J. L. MORENO AND THE PSYCHODRAMATIC METHOD

Beginning with a discussion of the intrinsic nature of psychodrama and providing the reader with a thorough description of the psychodramatic method, this book navigates the nature, applications, theories, and practices of the techniques originated by J. L. Moreno.

The book covers the work of the psychodrama pioneer in the field of mental health and discourse on his techniques. Methods of handling situations and scenarios that frequently arise in psychodrama sessions are described and amply illustrated with examples from actual psychodramas. The existential philosophy upon which psychodrama is founded, Moreno's Doctrine of Spontaneity-Creativity, and the theories important to understanding psychodrama are all discussed. The final chapter is devoted to the life and work of J. L. Moreno.

This book will be of great interest to psychodramatists, drama therapists, psychotherapists, and other mental health professionals who use the psychodramatic method in counseling and training programs.

John Nolte, PhD, has been a psychodramatic practitioner and trainer for more than 50 years. John has a doctorate in clinical psychology from Washington University and was trained in psychodrama by J. L. Moreno, MD, the originator of psychodrama and other action methods, and his wife, Zerka Moreno. He is certified as a Trainer-Educator-Practitioner by the American Board of Examiners in Psychodrama, Sociometry and Group Psychotherapy. He is recognized by the psychodrama community as a senior and respected practitioner of the Morenean methods as well as a seasoned trainer.

J. L. MORENO AND THE PSYCHODRAMATIC METHOD

On the Practice of Psychodrama

John Nolte

Routledge
Taylor & Francis Group
NEW YORK AND LONDON

First published 2020
by Routledge
52 Vanderbilt Avenue, New York, NY 10017

and by Routledge
2 Park Square, Milton Park, Abingdon, Oxon, OX14 4RN

Routledge is an imprint of the Taylor & Francis Group, an informa business

Library of Congress Cataloging-in-Publication Data
A catalog record for this book has been requested

ISBN: 978-0-367-22565-0 (hbk)
ISBN: 978-0-367-22566-7 (pbk)
ISBN: 978-0-429-27566-1 (ebk)

Typeset in Bembo
by Swales & Willis, Exeter, Devon, UK

To: Nancy Drew

CONTENTS

ACKNOWLEDGMENTS

I never miss a chance to express my deepest gratitude to J. L. and Zerka T. Moreno for all they have given to my personal and professional life. This book is another attempt to honor their gifts by passing them along. I hope others will appreciate everything they have bestowed upon the world.

Thanks to the American Society of Group Psychotherapy and Psychodrama and to President Nancy Kirsner for permission to include the Canon of Creativity in this book, as well as for the use of the illustration on the cover.

Marcia Hinckley, friend and English teacher, read much of the book and made a number of suggestions, many of which I gratefully incorporated.

Thanks also to John Ackerman, first for his brilliant inspiration to teach trial lawyers to be creative by introducing them to psychodrama, and then for his permission to use excerpts from his interview conducted so thoroughly by Dana Cole, another trial lawyer enthusiast.

I am deeply grateful to Gerry Spence, great American trial lawyer, who welcomed me in my attempt to introduce psychodrama into the teaching methods of his Trial Lawyers College. Neither of us anticipated how extensively we would find ways of integrating the method into the College or how creative students of the College would discover ways of using psychodrama in their everyday work. Working with trial lawyers, who deserve a far more favorable reputation than they have, has been one of the top experiences in my career. Spence has been a powerful advocate for psychodrama and I thank him for all he has contributed to the method and to me.

Don Clarkson, friend and colleague for many years, is responsible for my initial invitation to the Trial Lawyers College, and I cannot thank him too much for making that opportunity possible. Kätlin Larimer and Kathie St. Clair are the other two psychodramatists par excellence who made the

Trial Lawyers College so creative. They are also my partners in the National Psychodrama Training Center.

When Nancy Drew and I joined our lives together, I gained not only a wife and life partner but an outstanding editor as well. She bears much of the responsibility for the presence of this book. She encouraged me, sometimes forcefully, to get it done. She read everything that I wrote, including material that I wrote and then eliminated, and liberally used her red pencil to point out to me passages which needed work to make them intelligible. More importantly, with her grounding in philosophy, especially phenomenology and existentialism, she has helped me understand Moreno to a much greater extent. I hereby express my deepest appreciation to her.

INTRODUCTION

My first contact with psychodrama occurred early in my graduate student career when I came across a one-paragraph description in a textbook. As I recall, many years later, it declared that psychodrama was a method of psychotherapy devised by an Italian psychiatrist named Moreno, and consisted of patients performing skits based on their life experiences. I was not impressed. I was avidly reading my way through Freud's *Collected Works*, trying to make sense of psychoanalytic theory, and anticipating a career of practicing a psychodynamic style of psychotherapy. Performing skits seemed like a very superficial sort of psychotherapy. I was interested in a much more serious method.

I first encountered psychodrama in the fall of 1959, when a group from St. Louis State Hospital came to the Fulton (Missouri) State Hospital, where I was a staff clinical psychologist, to demonstrate the method. The presenters were all people I had known as a graduate student at Washington University in St. Louis: Abel Ossario, graduate school professor; Leon Fine, a fellow graduate student; and Barbara Seabourne, a fellow psychology trainee at John Cochran V. A. Hospital. I suspect that, still thinking of psychodrama in terms of the first description that I had read, I might not have attended the two-day demonstration of psychodrama had it not been presented by old friends.

The first session was a demonstration of spontaneity testing, not a classical psychodrama. However, I found it intriguing. After the session, I walked across the campus with my good friend, John Miller. We were in a very active discussion of what we had experienced, trying to figure out why the director had given the directions he had given, what the significance of the event was. Suddenly I stopped. "John," I said to my friend, "if psychodrama can get me this worked up, I think I need to find out more about it." I arranged to spend a few days at the St. Louis State Hospital with the psychodrama program headed by Leon Fine. Then, in the summer of 1962, I spent two weeks at the Moreno Institute. As psychodrama so often does to those who experience it, those two weeks changed the course of my life and I left committed to the psychodramatic method. It was also the first of many weeks I spent at the Institute, over a period of 14 years.

Since then, I have participated in at least five thousand psychodrama sessions as protagonist, director, auxiliary ego, training supervisor, and audience member. I have practiced psychodramatic psychotherapy in a state hospital and on psychiatric, substance abuse, and chronic pain services in several general hospitals, as well as in outpatient clinics. I have used psychodrama in organizational and staff development activities. I have employed role training with medical students and surgical residents and I have conducted in-service training sessions with nurses. I have utilized psychodrama in a university literature class. I have trained trial lawyers in trial skills and have made use of psychodrama in trial preparation. I have conducted training workshops in psychodrama for almost 50 years. I have served as Director of Training for the Moreno Institute.

I had a desire early in my psychodramatic career, while I was still very much a student of the method, to write about psychodrama, to write about spontaneity and warming up, surplus reality, role playing, and all the rest. I made many starts—but they all ended up way short of my goals and useless. What I didn't know then was that I didn't know nearly enough to articulate what I was learning and experiencing. I did write and co-write papers, some of which were published and some which were hand-outs for many presentations which I made at the Annual Conferences of the American Society of Group Psychotherapy and Psychodrama (ASGPP). A few years ago, I self-published them through Lulu.com as *The Psychodrama Papers*. When I finally got a "real" book thoroughly underway (Nolte, 2014), to the point that I thought I really could complete it, I discovered that it was turning out to be a book on J. L. Moreno's philosophy and theories. I added a section on methods as well. I also came to the realization that I was writing for discovery, to discover and put into words what I knew. I realized as well that this was what my first attempts to write about Moreno's ideas were about and that I simply did not have sufficient experience to accomplish what I wanted.

Several books whose titles suggest that there have been significant advances in psychodramatic theory, techniques, or practice, e.g. Holmes, Karp and Watson (1994); Gershoni (2003); Baim, Burmeister and Maciel (2007), have been published since Moreno's death in 1974. Although I do believe that the practice of psychodrama has changed since the Moreno Institute, representing the state of the art of psychodrama practice, ceased to exist, I am not convinced that practice has advanced. In fact, at the risk of being considered a troglodyte, I am of the opinion that psychodrama as generally practiced has suffered and is a less powerful method in the hands of many of today's psychodramatists than it was in Moreno's time. There are certainly exceptions to this statement. The practice of psychodrama presented in this book is the psychodramatic method as it was taught at the Moreno Institute in the 1960s and 1970s, the period during which I was associated with the Institute either as a student, staff member, or Director of Training. It reflects Zerka Moreno's style. I consider her my trainer, J. L. the originator. From him, I got the philosophy and theory. I am deeply and eternally grateful to both.

My hope is that those who read this book will find something in it that they did not already know, and that they will be glad that they learned. I expect that there will be readers who disagree with something that I have written. I will be disappointed if there are not. I would like to hear from all. Consider this, in Moreno's famous words, as my *Invitation to an Encounter.*

There are nine chapters in the book. The first five have to do with classical protagonist-centered psychodrama. This is psychodrama as it is employed for psychotherapy and for personal growth and development. The sixth chapter describes how psychodrama is and has been used for nonclinical objectives. Moreno was pained that his methods had often been adopted (and often modified), but separated from the theories and philosophy upon which they were based. Therefore, I would consider it amiss not to include a long chapter on Morenean theory, Chapter 7. Chapter 8 is a brief history of the psychodramatic method and Chapter 9 is my understanding of what J. L. Moreno was all about.

References

Baim, C., Burmeister, J. & Maciel, M. (Eds) (2007). *Psychodrama: Advances in Theory & Practice*. London: Routledge.

Gershoni, J. (Ed) (2003). *Psychodrama in the 21st Century: Clinical and Educational Applications*. New York: Springer..

Holmes, P., Karp, M. & Watson, M. (Eds) (1994). *Psychodrama since Moreno: Innovations in Theory and Practice*. London: Routledge.

Nolte, J. (2014). *The Philosophy, Theory and Methods of J. L. Moreno*. New York: Routledge.

1

WHAT IS PSYCHODRAMA, ANYWAY?

Role playing is a universal activity among children of all cultures. As children, we learn from older children or re-invent it ourselves. We teach school, explore outer space as astronauts, search for treasure buried by pirates, play doctor or cowboys and Indians, and engage in all sort of adventures. There are even suggestions that role playing is an evolutionary legacy from pre-human species. Philosophers, Rousseau, Froebel, and Dewey for example, had long pointed out that play was important in children's learning. It took the genius of J. L. Moreno, however, to transform the role-playing games of childhood into the organized, coherent, and structured method of psychodrama, that has since been employed in multiple ways, in education and training; in psychotherapy; in personal growth and development; and in social research.

More than a Method of Psychotherapy

The most common definition of psychodrama is based on its most widely applied function[1] as a method of psychotherapy, in which people act out the problematic situations in their current lives and troublesome ones from their past experiences instead of merely describing them as happens in conventional psychotherapies. The definition of psychodrama as a method of psychotherapy, however, greatly obscures the fact that it is a method which has several distinctly different applications. It is far more than just a psychotherapeutic method. In 1948, Ronald Levy wrote that in a broad general sense, psychodrama "includes the whole family of skills, techniques, and processes which are involved in the 'unrehearsed' but not unplanned, dramatization of human problems for the purpose of dealing with them more effectively" (p. 226).

Generically, psychodrama is a method of creating dramas, a systematized form of children's creative role playing. It is a *dramaturgy*, an art form. As such, it is also a *method of communication*. Psychodrama is a way to explore, understand, and express one's subjective experience, a *method of personality development*. Psychodrama is also a *method of training*, an *educational process*, and a *research instrument*. All these activities are legitimate functions of the psychodramatic method.

When he first offered training in his methods, psychodrama and sociometry, Moreno announced that his courses comprised educational, guidance, and marital counseling, mental disorders, and social maladjustment as subjects. The courses were open to educators, ministers, and counselors of all kinds, in addition to psychiatrists, social workers, and psychologists. It was clear that he saw psychodrama as far more than a psychotherapeutic method in the customary definition of medical psychiatry. The fact was that he saw therapy in a far broader sense than that of psychiatry. As a result, all students, whether counselors, therapists, teachers, or others, were taught the same thing—the basic psychodrama method. Moreno's concept of group psychotherapy as the therapy of the group rather than treatment of individuals in a group setting, and his mantra of "every person the therapist of every other person," were embedded in all the training at his Psychodramatic Institute.

A Dramaturgy

The lowest common denominator of psychodrama's functions is creating dramas. Every psychodrama, even if it is only a few minutes long, is indeed a dramatic piece. It is different from the conventional drama in that it does not require a script, trained actors, rehearsals, carefully constructed scenery, or costumes and props. In conventional theater, a proscenium arch separates the audience from the actors and the action. The psychodrama stage is easily accessible to the audience, from which come the protagonist and auxiliary players. A psychodrama is produced spontaneously in the moment, without a script, without rehearsals, scenery, and costumes, and with a minimum of props. The protagonist and actors emerge from the audience and return to it. Rather than to interpret an author's work, the role of the director is to assist the protagonist to communicate her or his subjective experiences in dramatic form. That psychodrama is a dramaturgy also means that psychodrama is an art form.

A Method of Communication

There are many wonderful definitions of art (Popova, 2012). One of my favorites is: "A work of art is a message to the world, from the world, about the world."[2] Psychodrama is without question a method of communication. It provides a unique and powerful way to convey to others what we have experienced in our lives. The audience is invited to be present as we recreate and act out events and fantasies complete with our thoughts and our feelings. In psychodrama, the protagonist doesn't tell a story from his or her life. He or she *re-lives* an experience, a wish, a dream, or a fantasy in the presence of the audience. In the process, the actions, interactions, thoughts, and emotions of the protagonist and of all the other individuals involved are portrayed in a richness, intensity, depth, vibrancy, and completeness that goes far beyond narrative. We observe and participate in the protagonist's tribulation, pain, joy, triumph, and celebration. We see the protagonist and his or her life as the protagonist experiences it.

The most important communication is the protagonist's communication with him or herself. Through reenactment of experiences, the protagonist extracts information that has remained hidden and inaccessible. The protagonist thus comes to know her or himself more thoroughly. Through psychodrama, one makes sense out of events that have heretofore been confusing, baffling, perplexing, or bewildering.

A Method of Psychotherapy

The most extensive application of psychodrama has been in the mental health field. This is not surprising since Moreno was a psychiatrist who first employed spontaneity drama techniques to resolve troubles in a distressed marriage in the early 1920s. Moreno developed the psychotherapeutic function of psychodrama in conjunction with his establishment of a psychiatric hospital, Beacon Hill Sanitarium in Beacon, NY, in 1936. The protagonists of the early psychodramas were psychiatric patients. Psychodrama, with its emphasis upon interpersonal relationships, reflected Moreno's conviction that psychiatric symptoms result from interpersonal problems rather than from internal conflicts. This was contrary to the conventional viewpoint, the medical model of mental illness. For Moreno, treatment was focused on relationships, groups, and society at large.

Psychodrama is uniquely designed to achieve what psychotherapy seeks to do, i.e., to provide relief from emotional distress. By replicating direct experience in a flexible and controlled setting, psychodrama provides deep insight into the genesis of one's actions. The action insight that the protagonist earns from psychodramatic work is deeper and far more effective than the cognitive insight a client receives from conventional psychotherapy.

Personality Development

"Know thyself," the famous Greek aphorism often attributed to Socrates, has elicited similar points of view over the centuries, for example:

> I must first know myself, as the Delphian inscription says; to be curious about that which is not my concern, while I am still in ignorance of my own self would be ridiculous.
>
> *Plato*

> He who knows others is wise; he who knows himself is enlightened.
>
> *Lao Tzu*

> Make it thy business to know thyself, which is the most difficult lesson in the world.
>
> *Miguel de Cervantes*

> Observe all men; thy self most.
>
> *Benjamin Franklin*

Other expressions incorporating the notion of self knowledge with an emphasis on being include:

> "Know Thyself" was written over the portal of the antique world. Over the portal of the new world, "Be Thyself" shall be written.
>
> *Oscar Wilde*

> We only become what we are by the radical and deep-seated refusal of that which others have made of us.
>
> *Jean-Paul Sartre*

> Without self knowledge, without understanding the working and functions of his machine, man cannot be free, he cannot govern himself and he will always remain a slave.
>
> *G. I. Gurdjieff*

Psychodrama reflects the spirit of all of these views.

Expanded understanding of oneself, insight, is a basic principle of most methods of psychotherapy. However, one need not have a psychiatric problem to desire, seek, and benefit from greater self awareness and self understanding. Moreno sometimes described psychodrama as therapy for normal people.[3] Psychodrama is a powerful method for the re-examination of one's life experiences, especially those that are associated with strong positive or negative emotion. Highly functional people find value in participating in activities that generate insight. These include psychotherapies of many kinds, personal growth and development groups, and psychodrama training groups where people have opportunities for exploring puzzling and problematic events in their lives. Psychodrama, which involves the whole person physically, mentally, and socially, is the most powerful approach to the task of greater self understanding.

For several decades in the last half of the twentieth century, the human potential movement consisted of a wide variety of workshops often labeled as human skills training, personal growth and development workshops, or as encounter groups. These events made use of psychotherapeutic techniques as well as techniques developed from small group research. They promised increased personal effectiveness. Jonathan Moreno (2014) discusses the history of the human potential movement and its relationship to the theory and methods of J. L. Moreno at length in his book about his father. The psychodrama training workshops of the Moreno Institute provided a prototype for these events. Personal growth activities are differentiated from psychotherapy in that the latter is considered remedial, treatment of a disorder, while the former involves expansion of self understanding and social effectiveness.

Social Skills or Role Training

One of the earliest nonclinical applications of psychodrama was role training, a form of psychodrama that prepares a person to meet future situations. Role training allows one to experience anticipated difficult situations on the psychodrama stage and to practice responding to them in a safe setting. Psychodramatic techniques were used for training as early as 1928 when Moreno conducted role training sessions for managers of Macy's Department Store (J. D. Moreno, 2014). A few years later, Moreno was deeply immersed in his pioneering sociometric research project at the New York Training School for Girls at Hudson. One of the problems he confronted was preparing students for successful living in open society after discharge from the institution. In the first edition of *Who Shall Survive?* Moreno (1934) describes role-playing sessions in which the students of the New York State Training School for Girls were put in situations that they might expect to experience after leaving the institution. Since then, role training or some modification of it has found widespread usage in many venues and especially in business and industrial situations where it is often referred to as role play. Moreno sometimes called role training "rehearsal for living."

Noted industrial psychologist Norman R. F. Maier made extensive use of psychodramatic role playing in the business world. Maier worked with large industries on the problems of improving supervision. The program was focused on moving leadership from an autocratic model to a more democratic one. In his books (1952, 1953, 1955) Maier describes many ways in which role playing can be used to introduce human relations training into the industrial setting.

Psychodrama in Education

Psychodrama has been creatively employed by teachers and instructors in many disciplines. In literature, for example, a class turns a discussion into dramatic form. Narrative is enacted. Students take the roles of characters, expanding on the roles and answering questions that other class members may have. A systematic approach to psychodramatization of literary works is called bibliodrama and has been written about by Miller (1998, 2000, 2002; Pitzele, 1998).

The first article in the journal, *Sociometry*, documenting the use of a psychodrama in a formal teaching setting, appeared in 1939 when J. G. Franz of Columbia University reported using spontaneity training with students in a public speaking course. The first book on Morenean methods in the field of education, *Psychodrama and Sociometry in American Education*, was published in 1949 (Haas). It consisted of more than 30 articles by as many authors describing a wide range of applications from early elementary grades through junior high school, high school, and college levels to community projects.

Since 1934, there have been dozens, if not hundreds of articles in professional journals and books describing or advocating the use of psychodrama for teaching. In addition to the term psychodrama, the authors of these papers have used the labels sociodrama, spontaneity training, role training, simulations, and role playing in describing the use of spontaneity methods for teaching an exceptionally wide range of subjects. A cursory search of the JSTOR archive resulted in papers reporting the use of the spontaneity drama in method in more than 25 different subjects ranging from aesthetics and accounting through history and literature to philosophy and sociology. The creativity of the teachers who designed these events is awe-inspiring. Teachers who have written about role playing experiences are enthusiastic about the method. The number of events reported in professional journals is probably an infinitesimally small percentage of the total number of role playing events in the classroom.

Research

Because it highlights social interaction, psychodrama and its sibling method, sociodrama, provide a unique method for conducting social research. Reenactment methods have been extensively used in social psychological research. A modification of psychodrama, reenactment interviewing, has been successfully applied to qualitative research (Drew, 1993). Research is a greatly underused function of psychodrama.

The Current Status of Psychodrama

Psychodrama has never achieved the popularity in the mental health field in America to which its effectiveness entitles it. The number of certified psychodramatists has remained between 400 and 450 for some years, although the number of actual practitioners may be twice that. In addition, many practitioners of other methods include psychodramatic interventions in their work. On the other hand, psychodrama has found popularity in South American countries, especially Argentina and Brazil where estimates run as high as 6,000 psychodramatists. The same is true in Europe where there are training programs and practitioners of the method in many countries.

Notes

1 I first heard Jim Enneis, founder and long-time director of the Psychodrama Training Program of St. Elizabeth Hospital, use the term, *function*, for the different applications of psychodrama. Considering its dictionary definition as "the action for which a person or thing is specially fitted or used or for which a thing exists," it seems a very appropriate word in this context.

2 From Matt Parrish, a good friend who was himself an artist and musician as well as a great psychiatrist. I do not know if it is original with him but suspect that it is.

3 The number of self-help books in print indicates that there is an extensive feeling among people that they are not as effective as they wish or think that they should be. The human potential movement, also known as the encounter group movement, was a response to that feeling.

References

Drew, N. (1993). Reenactment interviewing: a methodology for phenomenological research. *Image – The Journal of Nursing Scholarship*, 25, 345–351.

Franz, J. G. (1939). Spontaneity training in public speaking classes: a preliminary report. *Sociometry*, 2, 49–53.

Haas, R. B. (Ed.) (1949). *Psychodrama and Sociodrama in American Education*. Beacon, NY: Beacon House.

Levy, R. (1948). Psychodrama and the philosophy of cultural education. *Sociatry*, 2, 225–234.

Maier, N. (1952). *Principles of human relations: applications to management*. New York: John Wiley & Sons.

Maier, N. (1953). Dramatized case material as a springboard for role playing. *Group Psychotherapy*, 6, 30–42.

Maier, N. (1955). *A psychological approach to industrial problems*. Boston, MA: Houghton Mifflin.

Miller, D. (1998). *Doers of the world: how stories come to life through bibliodrama*. Redlands, CA: Beacon Book Remainders.

Miller, D. (2000). *Parables of Jesus: a creative resource for bibliodrama*. Redlands, CA: Beacon Book Remainders.

Miller, D. (2002). *Bibliodrama of Job*. Redlands, CA: Beacon Book Remainders Psychodramas.

Moreno, J. D. (2014). *Impromptu man*. New York: Bellevue Literary Press.

Moreno, J. L. (1934). *Who shall survive? A new approach to the problems of human interrelations.* Washington, DC: Nervous and Mental Disease Publishing Company.

Pitzele, P. (1998). *Scripture windows: toward a practice of bibliodrama.* Los Angeles, CA: Torah Aura.

Popova, M. (2012). What is art? www.brainpickings.org/2012/06/22/what-is-art/, accessed December 5, 2017.

2

THE BASICS OF PSYCHODRAMA

J. L. Moreno read a short paper, an introduction to psychodrama, at the American Psychiatric Association's annual conference in 1946. He published the four-page document later that year in *Sociometry* (1946a), and a reprint of it was given to every visitor to the Moreno Institute thereafter. The three phases and five instruments of psychodrama as laid out in that work have been repeated in almost every explication of psychodrama since, including the present one.

The Three Phases of a Psychodrama Session

A psychodrama session consists of three parts or phases. The first is the warming up phase. Warming up is a very important concept in spontaneity–creativity work. The next chapter is dedicated to an exploration of warming up and the warming up phase of a psychodrama session. The warming up phase is followed by the action phase, the drama proper. This is a co-production of the director and protagonist, assisted by other group members as auxiliary egos. The action phase of a psychodrama session will also be explored in its own chapter. The final phase is called sharing and involves group members revealing how their life experiences connect with those portrayed by the protagonist. Sharing plays a significant role in why this is a group method even though a classical psychodrama is centered on a single individual.

The Five Instruments of Psychodrama

Moreno identified five components of psychodrama which he called the instruments of psychodrama. They are: the stage; the protagonist, the director, auxiliary egos, usually simply called auxiliaries, and the audience or group. The psychodrama, Moreno wrote, is co-created by the director and protagonist. A psychodrama unfolds a story of which the protagonist is the hero.

The Stage

The first instrument of psychodrama is the stage. A stage is a magical space, especially a psychodrama stage. We can conjure up any place on this stage, real or imaginary, that the protagonist desires or needs to visit and experience. Heaven, Hell, outer space, or inner space are no problem for the psychodrama stage. We can call anybody alive, dead, or imaginary with whom the protagonist desires or needs to interact to this stage. If that individual is absent, dead, or imaginary, psychodrama can, none the less, give them a physical form via an auxiliary ego. No proscenium separates the psychodrama stage from the audience space. There is no backstage. Everything occurs in the open. Protagonist and auxiliary egos can move easily from audience to stage and back into the audience again. The formal psychodrama stage is round and has several levels. Children immediately recognize and embrace the magic of the psychodrama stage; on entering a psychodrama theater, their first impulse is to run up on the accessible stage, ready to act out their fantasies. Adults are often similarly tempted but may not be so bold.

The stage, Moreno says, offers us a flexible and multi-dimensional living space, unlike the narrow and restraining living space of reality. "The stage space is an extension of life beyond the reality tests of life itself. Reality and fantasy are not in conflict, but both are functions within a wider sphere—the psychodramatic world of objects, persons and events" (p. 249). The stage provides freedom to experience and express oneself.

Moreno, through the good offices of Gertrude Franchot Tone, constructed a theater especially designed for psychodrama when he acquired the property that became Beacon Hill Sanitarium. Built in what was originally the carriage house, it featured a circular stage of three levels. In addition, a balcony partially supported by two columns from the stage furnished a fourth level. Two battens of conventional stage lights in the ceiling lighted both the lower stage and the balcony. Stage lights provided red, blue, and amber lights as well as white bulbs and the wiring was such that colors could be adjusted separately for both intensity and hue. Thus, the stage could be bathed in a deep blue light to emphasize a protagonist's sorrow, or in red to underscore anger. A similar stage, elliptical instead of round, was built in the New York City Moreno Institute. There have been a few other psychodrama theaters constructed in various locations, St. Elizabeth Hospital in Washington, D. C., Harvard University, St. Louis State Hospital, for example. I built a small psychodrama theater in Indianapolis that was in use for the ten years that I lived there and for a few years later. However, only a small percent of psychodramas are ever produced on stages especially built for the purpose. By far the vast number of psychodramas are created in ordinary rooms or offices, and the stage is simply a space in the middle or at one end of the room that is so designated. It is any space in which psychodramatic action takes place.

An assigned stage area is important for it identifies a space that can become any place that the protagonist chooses, once the action part of a session begins. It is the space in which the protagonist is allowed everything necessary to produce the his or her inner subjectivity. On stage, surplus reality reigns. Group members assigned auxiliary roles put their spontaneity and themselves in service to the protagonist's needs, taking and playing roles according to the protagonist's specifications. Off the stage, the group members who have been auxiliary egos relate to the protagonist with their own perceptions and feelings. It is especially important for protagonists who are delusional to have an appointed space in which the delusion can be acted out and lived, separated from the space in which the realities of ordinary life prevail.

The Protagonist

People who are offered the role of protagonist in a psychodrama session for the first time often respond, "I can't act!" That, of course, is not a problem. Protagonists are only asked to act themselves, to portray their everyday lives as well as their private thoughts and feelings. The protagonist is invited to act freely whatever comes to mind, and is given freedom of expression to do so. The aim is to go beyond verbal description by putting thoughts and feelings into action, to act them out. A psychodrama mantra is "Don't tell me. *Show* me."

Most psychodrama sessions are created from the life events, emotions, dreams, fantasies, ambitions, or anticipations of the future of the protagonist. The majority of psychodramas in both therapy groups and personal growth and development groups begin with some sort of problem or question that perturbs the protagonist. A disturbing thought, uncomfortable feelings like anxiety, depression, anger and fear, acting in ways that one recognizes as self-defeating, rejection by a friend, a mystifying response from a significant other, a disturbing dream, and concern about the future are common starting points for psychodramas. Almost always there is a puzzle or a question to be answered.

Actually there is no requirement for there to be a problem. Moreno often said that one could profit from psychodramatizing every truly meaningful experience, positive or negative, that there was something to be learned from both kinds. I made use of this notion when I found myself invited to present on psychodrama to civic groups, like mental health associations. Living in the Midwest and uncomfortable with the public sessions such as were offered in New York where protagonists dealt with the same kind of issues as in therapy or personal growth groups, I chose to warm my public groups up to meaningful experiences. Then I could choose a positive one and create the drama with a willing protagonist without a problem (Nolte, 2008). Since then I have used the psychodramatization of meaningful experiences as an exercise for novice directors in training groups. The fact that there is no problem to be resolved reduces the anxiety that often accompanies early attempts to direct psychodrama.

In a psychodrama, the subjective world of the protagonist, how one perceives one's world and others in it, what one thinks and feels, one's ambitions, desires, and fears, and everything that ordinarily goes on internally and invisibly, is acted out, externalized and made visible by being produced on the psychodramatic stage. The major responsibility of the protagonist is to be truthful. Moreno (1946a) wrote, "Psychodrama can be defined, therefore, as the science which explores the 'truth' by dramatic methods" (p. 249). The word "truth" is set in quotation marks to signify that Moreno meant the protagonist's subjective truth. This is existential truth rather than historic fact. This truth is the truth as one knows it, the truth that a witness in a courtroom swears to tell, one's conviction of what one has observed and experienced. Acting out one's truth is seldom a burden on a protagonist. Most protagonists are searching for greater understanding of their inner worlds, seeking for the truth of their interactions with others. Many protagonists confirm that the role of protagonist on the psychodrama stage encourages one to be honest. Even committed schizophrenic patients, convinced that they are not in need of treatment, who may initially resist becoming protagonists find great satisfaction in portraying their perceptions of their psychotic worlds, the truth as they know it (J. L. Moreno, 1940, 1944, 1959). The goal of psychodrama is not to produce actors in the conventional sense of theatrical actors but to encourage individuals to be that which they truly are, often more completely than they have been able to achieve in their lives.

The Director

The third instrument of psychodrama is the director. The initial role of the director is that of the dramaturge. It is the director's responsibility to create a drama with the content presented by the protagonist. The psychodrama is a co-creation of the director and the protagonist, according to Moreno. A psychodrama can be produced with only the first three instruments, the protagonist, the director, and a space or stage on which to work.

Directing psychodrama is an extraordinarily complex process. Karp (1998) lists two dozen directorial tasks. The director has first to be familiar with the techniques of the psychodramatic method. More important than the techniques themselves is learning how to use them effectively to present the subjective thoughts and feelings of the protagonist in the form of a drama. This means learning when to call for a role reversal, when to ask the protagonist to soliloquize, and when to stage a mirror, for example. Directing skill includes the ability to assist the protagonist in identifying emotions that may not be immediately clear, even to the protagonist. The director's resources for accomplishing the primary task include the sensitivity to consistently assess the protagonist's warming up process and the director's own spontaneity. The director who has a talent for storytelling and a sense of the dramatic will more consistently direct dramas that are aesthetically satisfying to the protagonist and group members, as well as being beneficial for both. Competency as a director requires both extensive training, experience, and deep-seated self understanding.

Adding to the complexity of creating a drama, the director has one or more additional roles that are related to the purpose of the psychodrama session. If the psychodrama is conducted, for example, as psychotherapy or group therapy session, the director's additional role is that of psychotherapist. If the purpose is training, the director is a trainer in addition to being a psychodramatist. If the psychodrama session is conducted in a substance abuse program, the director must also be a substance abuse counselor. If it involves a lawyer, a lawsuit, or a lawyer's client, the director is a trial consultant in addition to being a director. In each event, the psychodrama director must have some professional competence or expertise in addition to psychodrama directing skills. Once the ability to consistently produce a successful psychodrama is acquired, one can develop ways of modifying and applying the psychodrama method to problems in almost any area involving interpersonal interaction.

The Auxiliary Ego

As noted earlier, individuals in this role are usually called auxiliaries rather than auxiliary egos. "Ego" is used here in the philosophical sense of a conscious, thinking subject, rather than in the psychoanalytic notion as a part of the mind. Moreno used the term to underscore his conviction of the interpersonal nature of most emotional problems. The use of auxiliaries to engage with the protagonist differentiates psychodrama from psychotherapeutic methods that perceive one's problems as belonging to oneself. For Moreno, the problems we encounter in life involve other people, individuals who are as sentient, willful, and spontaneous as ourselves are. Moreno had noted during his work with the spontaneity theater which he directed in Vienna in the 1920s, that individuals on stage by themselves could freely improvise with little difficulty. This ability changed drastically when a second player was introduced and the two had to collaborate in creating a dramatic piece—just as happens in real life. The auxiliary ego is to be understood as a helping or supporting other person who makes it possible for the protagonist to explore his or her relationships with the other important people in her or his life.

The first responsibility of the auxiliary is to take an assigned role and interact with the protagonist in that role. The role most frequently is that of an absent significant other, someone who may be either alive or dead. The auxiliary may also play a role that exists only in the imagination of protagonist or the role of a pet, a dog or cat for example, and even an inanimate object such as a picture on a wall. In the therapy of psychotic individuals, the auxiliary may be asked to play an hallucination or delusion. Finally, auxiliaries also play an aspect or part of the protagonist's self or an emotion, the protagonist's fear, anger, or courage, perhaps.

The second responsibility of the auxiliary is to approximate as closely as possible the protagonist's perception of the role that the auxiliary takes, which enhances the protagonist's spontaneity and allows him or her to experience more fully the emotions that exist between the protagonist and the significant other. The auxiliary can advance the drama by matching the protagonist's emotional intensity and taking some freedom for spontaneous interaction with the protagonist, always remaining in the role of the significant other. Faced with a question or confrontation for which the response is not clear, the auxiliary can utilize his or her own feelings to respond. Often enough, the auxiliary's response is accurate and adequate to the situation. If it is not, it is a small matter to correct the response with a simple role reversal that gives the auxiliary more information about the role of the significant other.

Having successfully accomplished these basic functions, the auxiliary assists the director investigate the relationship between the protagonist and the significant other. Auxiliaries achieve this by being aware and then expressing the feelings that are aroused in them by interaction with the protagonist. Because we are all more alike than we are different, our emotional responses to a given situation are similar even in role playing. In addition, we find quite often that the individuals chosen for auxiliary roles have life experiences that connect them with the roles for which they have been chosen. This happens too often to be a chance effect and is explained by the Morenean concept of tele, a concept that will be discussed in a later chapter on psychodramatic theory. These connections between auxiliaries and their assigned roles are usually discovered during the sharing phase of psychodrama.

Auxiliaries who trust their spontaneity are often quite accurate in their portrayals of the significant other. When they are accurate, they enhance the dramatic aspects of psychodrama. Good auxiliary work can increase the protagonist's perception of the significant other—even though the auxiliary has never met that person. Auxiliaries' understanding of the roles they are called on to play can be expressed in the drama itself, as well as in sharing at the conclusion of action.

Although most people can play auxiliary roles effectively, skill is involved and this skill can be learned and increased. Some people are naturally adept at putting themselves into the roles of others. Everybody has some awareness and knowledge of most, if not all, the roles in their own culture. Even six and seven year old children are capable of producing recognizable enactments or description of many common roles in their culture.

Being frequently picked to play roles in psychodrama develops skill as an auxiliary. Hence, individuals with a lot of psychodramatic experience tend to be more active and have greater trust in their spontaneity while serving as auxiliaries. In training groups we find that group members often seek auxiliary roles. They like becoming part of the action and recognize that their participation is a gift to the protagonist. Once one gets over the shock of being picked to play negative roles, as I experienced when asked early in my training to play the role of an adolescent brother who attempted to rape his younger sister, group members often relish taking "bad guy" roles. When a group member expresses anxiety about being selected to take a negative role, the protagonist can be asked to explain why this particular individual was chosen for this particular role. The protagonist's answer invariably includes a statement of trust in the chosen individual. We don't choose someone that we don't trust to play an abuser in our psychodramas.

My opinion is that playing the roles of abusing parents, tyrannical bosses, rapists, and the like allows us to experience roles that we reject in our lives. In other words, it gives us the opportunity to encounter and express our shadow self.

Moreno described the auxiliary as an extension of both the protagonist and the director. Directors must maintain a high level of objectivity to ensure that their own subjective feelings do not intrude into the drama. As it is sometimes expressed, directors must bracket their feelings. Auxiliaries are allowed to express the emotions they experience in role vis-à-vis the protagonist. The assumption is that what the auxiliary feels is in response to the protagonist and belongs to the role the auxiliary is playing. If personal feelings intrude into the auxiliary's portray of the significant other, the director has ways for correcting the auxiliary's representation. In the process of engaging with the protagonist, the auxiliary is exploring the relationship of the protagonist and significant other, providing information and cues for the director.

In the early years of psychodrama, Moreno used trained members of his staff as auxiliaries. When he called for a role reversal, he expected auxiliaries to assume the other role while changing places with the protagonist, and to immediately repeat the last phrase or sentence spoken by the protagonist. The purpose was to keep the action flowing as smoothly as possible. Today's psychodramatists, aware of the salutary effect of being an auxiliary, usually allow protagonists to choose auxiliaries from among the group members to play the roles of absent significant others. A few directors prefer to use a team of trained individuals (see Hudgens, 2002, for example).

The Group

With the exception of psychodrama *a deux*, Moreno's term for a psychodramatist working with a client alone, psychodrama is ordinarily conducted in the context of a group. In a single psychodrama session, there is customarily one protagonist and a single psychodrama, although in some psychodramatic therapy groups several members may engage in shorter psychodramatic pieces. At first glance, this makes psychodrama appear to be individual psychotherapy in a group setting rather than group therapy, a practice of which that Moreno was critical. In his concept of social psychiatry (or sociatry), Moreno considered group therapy to be therapy of the group. Participation in a few psychodrama sessions makes it quite clear that group members in addition to the protagonist profit from the drama. First of all, there is the phenomenon of audience catharsis, identified by Aristotle. Group members invariably become emotionally involved in a competently directed psychodrama, often identifying with the protagonist or another individual in the psychodrama. It is not unusual for group members to gain a new understanding of their own relationships, a catharsis of integration, while watching a protagonist struggle with theirs. There is also benefit discussed above that comes from becoming an auxiliary in the drama. As pointed out above, auxiliaries often discover that they have a significant relationship with the roles for which they are picked. The experience may give them new insights into themselves. The sharing phase of the session allows an opportunity for the group to reveal the impact of the drama on the group members and to identify their connections to each other as well as to the protagonist.

The group is important in other ways, too. As a social entity, it is representative of the culture in which the group was formed. Thus it reflects that culture's values and stands for public opinion. In group-centered psychodrama, the protagonist emerges from the group and portrays a problem common to the group. This allows the group to proceed to the next common issue.

The sociometry of the group plays a role, often extremely subtle, in the selection of a protagonist and in the theme of the psychodrama. When a group comes together, there are a variety of positive and negative reactions of the members for each other. These reactions include both transference and tele. That is to say, they are based on both accurate and inaccurate perceptions of each other. Regardless, these feelings strongly and subtly influence the warming up process of the group and the selection of the protagonist.

Psychodrama Techniques

Psychodrama techniques are the instructions or directions that the director gives to the protagonist and auxiliaries in the process of creating a drama. They are designed to turn inner subjectivity into external action. Moreno (1958) reported that a co-worker had counted 350 different psychodramatic techniques. Few practicing psychodramatists today would attempt to list more than a dozen or so. The psychodramatic literature contains many discussions of techniques and each listing is a little different from the others. Five or six techniques, commonly involved in psychodramatic production show up in most listings. One or more other techniques are frequently included. Often listed as techniques are some procedures that actually involve a combination of basic techniques. Dream psychodrama, future projection, or decision making are examples. I prefer to think of these commonly used structures as conventions, combinations of techniques that have been found helpful for psychodramatizing situations that frequently occur in psychodramas. In addition to techniques and conventions there are combinations of psychodrama with other methods such as hypnosis. Zerka Moreno (1965) called these adjunct methods.

A baker's dozen of psychodramatic techniques that I consider to be the most basic ones are described in this chapter. These include the initial interview; self presentation; scene setting; soliloquy; role reversal; doubling; encounter; mirror; the empty chair; director's confrontation; concretization; improvisation, and matryoshka doll. The more complex combinations of techniques and adjunct methods will be discussed in Chapter 4 on Creating a Drama.

Initial Interview

A protagonist has been selected and it is time for the action session, for the drama to begin. Psychodramas most commonly start with an initial interview. The initial interview can accomplish several tasks. It serves to warm the individual up to the role of protagonist if the group warming up process and selection of the protagonist have not been sufficient to do so. The initial interview can also be used to slow down protagonists who are overly warmed up to their issues or to a particular event. The initial interview can also clarify the issues and, if necessary, a contract between the director and protagonist can be struck.

The initial interview does not have to be very long. Moreno exhorted directors to avoid letting the protagonist tell the story in lieu of dramatizing it. Once the first scene or starting point of the protagonist is identified, the interview can be considered to have accomplished its purpose and the drama can get underway. The content of the drama unfolds from there on in action.

Here is an example of a brief initial interview followed by getting the information in action. The drama takes place in a training group and the protagonist is a woman in her mid-30s, familiar with the psychodramatic method, who has already stated that she wants to explore unsettling and depressive feelings she had after a recent visit to the town from which she had moved not too long ago.

DIRECTOR: You've had these feelings since you visited your old hometown?

PROTAGONIST: Yes.

DIRECTOR: We need a place to begin. Do you have an idea or could we go to the moment you decided to make the visit?

PROTAGONIST: That sounds good to me.

DIRECTOR: It will help us understand the situation, I think. Where are we when you decide to visit. Take us there. *(The protagonist sets the scene of her living room. The director helps by asking a few questions about the scene. It is in the evening. Her two dogs are with her.)* Soliloquize.

PROTAGONIST: I've been living here for six months and haven't really made any friends. It's my birthday next weekend and I really don't have anybody I want to help me celebrate. *(Etc. Then:)* Why don't I go back to Springfield for my birthday where I've got family to celebrate with?

DIRECTOR: Fine. Is there anything we need to see before we go back?

PROTAGONIST: *(Thinking.)* I don't believe so. Wait! There's a telephone call with my mother.

DIRECTOR: O.K. Let's see that. Where are you when you have this call?

(Scene is set.)

In this brief fragment of a psychodrama, the interview is very short. The protagonist is quite experienced with psychodrama and she and the director have created dramas together several times. This familiarity with each other and the trust between them makes is easy to get into action early. In setting the scene, the protagonist is in psychodramatic action. The next direction is a soliloquy in which the content of the drama begins to be produced. This is getting it in action rather than through interview.

Sometimes, as here, what starts out to be an initial scene reveals that there is an earlier event which is integral to the protagonist's story. This doesn't really cause a problem. We simply go to the new initial scene. Psychodrama is, if one allows it to be, a very flexible instrument. In nautical terms, it is a forgiving craft; mistakes and missteps are easily corrected.

Self Presentation

Moreno calls this the simplest psychodramatic technique (1937, p. 26). The protagonist enacts situations which are representative of the protagonist's daily life. The protagonist also enacts and presents as accurately and thoroughly as possible the other people who are in the protagonist's life. Everybody has a number of roles in life. What is referred to as one's self is, in Morenean theory, one's role repertoire, the roles in which one functions in daily life. Moreno's role theory is the source of this notion and is discussed in the chapter on psychodrama theory. It is sufficient here to say that we act (and often look) differently from one role to another. The judge on the bench hearing a criminal case behaves differently than the same individual in the role of father playing ball with his ten year old son, or reading a story to her daughter, even though both roles make use of the same physical body. In self presentation, protagonists present one or more of the roles in which they function. Moreno frequently began psychodramas by asking protagonists to show the group a common activity which they frequently carried out in everyday life. By doing so, he gave an anxious protagonist an easy task with which to warm up to action and also provided the group with an opportunity to see the protagonist in a daily life situation. The protagonist in the psychodramatic fragment above first presents herself as a newcomer without many connections in her new community. Later in the drama, she acts out her roles of a daughter, of a close friend, and an ex-lover.

Self presentation also includes the presentation of significant others who are necessary for reenactment of scenes in the protagonist's life. Their roles are taken by group members serving as auxiliaries but first the protagonist in role reversal shows the auxiliary and the group how they look and act, as the protagonist perceives them. The procedure is explained in some detail in the section on role reversal.

Scene Setting

The impossibility of knowing ahead of time what the scenes of a psychodrama will be or where the psychodrama will take us precludes the use of scenery and other than simple props. Again we can think of childhood role playing games where a closed fist with a pointed index finger becomes a deadly revolver or a cardboard box a trusty spaceship. The wonderful technical stagecraft of the conventional theater is not available to the psychodramatist. The psychodrama director makes up for that with scene setting technique. Once the protagonist has identified an event or experience to be enacted, the director asks first, "Where does this take place?" and then, "Set the scene. Show us what it is like here." The protagonist is then assisted by questions from the director to give a detailed description of the setting in which the action takes place. If the scene is in a room indoors, the director will want to know the size of the room, the nature of the floor ("Is the floor carpeted or bare?"), the walls ("Painted? Papered? What color?"), how the room is lighted, where are doors and windows, what is in the room and where located, etc. The director considers all the senses and may ask about the temperature, perhaps the texture of a wall or item in the room, the aromas we smell (particularly if the scene is characterized by smells, like a kitchen), the sounds that we hear in this place, and so forth. Many directors begin scene setting of a room by asking the protagonist to locate a door into the room somewhere on stage, then to stand in the door way and, "Describe what we would see if we were standing here with you." As the protagonist identifies items in the room, chairs, table, the TV, the stove, or refrigerator, the director encourages them to move around the room and identify the location of these things, using chairs, small tables, cushions, or whatever is available, sometimes simply imagination.

Scene setting accomplishes several things that enhance the drama for both protagonists and group members. Setting the scene serves to warm the protagonist up to the situation that is to be dramatized. This effect is especially marked when the scene is from the distant past. Protagonists recall much more about a scene when they are moving about in the space of the stage, signifying items, their description, and location than when they are simply describing the same scene in words only.

It is clear to the experience psychodramatist that memory is not simply a neurological function. Memory is neuro-muscular.

In addition to warming protagonists up to scenes, scene setting warms the group members up to the protagonist as well as to the scene. Just as we learn much about new acquaintances when we are invited into their homes, we learn about protagonists when they invite us into their personal spaces. As the protagonist moves about the stage, points out furniture and objects that we cannot actually see, we form pictures in our minds. The scene becomes real not only for the protagonist but for group members as well. When people recall the psychodrama of another person, they typically recall the scene which the protagonist set. In a sense, psychodrama results in a shared hallucination.

Soliloquy

Soliloquy is a technique that has been widely utilized in conserve theater, the tactic that great playwrights like Shakespeare employed, many of which have become widely known and famous. Hamlet's "To be or not to be" speech, and Jacque's "All the world's a stage" are examples. Playwrights use soliloquy when it is important for the audience to know the innermost thoughts of a character. Psychodrama directors make use of it in the same way. Soliloquy reveals the internal, subjective thoughts and feelings of the protagonist, making them open and available. It is especially helpful when a protagonist is face to face with a significant other, such as a parent or a supervisor, expressing one feeling and suppressing a very different one. Here is an example:

The protagonist is reenacting a childhood scene. She is the oldest of three sisters in a chaotic family. In this scene she has just interrupted a screaming match between her mother and the next younger sister.

DIRECTOR: So they stop fighting. What happens now?

PROTAGONIST: I am in the living room with mother. I am crying and she is comforting me while I cry. *(The protagonist kneels with her head in mother's lap and her mother is stroking her hair. Protagonist indicates that the auxiliary is not accurate.)*

DIRECTOR: Reverse roles and show us how mother is.

"MOTHER" (P): You are the only one who understands me. I don't know what I would do without you. You are the only one I like. I don't like either of your sisters.

DIRECTOR: Reverse back. *(Protagonist assumes her own role. The auxiliary mother repeats the words. The protagonist sobs in her mother's lap but does not say anything.)* Soliloquize. What are you thinking and feeling?

PROTAGONIST: Here I am again, crying in the lap of this woman, my mother, when I really hate her. She is not a mother. She is awful. I wish I could trade her in for a new model. I do this to get mother's attention off my little sister.

Another major application of soliloquy is to assist protagonists to sort out and identify feelings that have often been denied, suppressed, or repressed. *In the psychodrama, the protagonist confronts a friend whom she has told in confidence but who has revealed to another acquaintance that the protagonist has had a miscarriage.*

PROTAGONIST: I am really hurt. I told you about the miscarriage in confidence. I said that I didn't want a lot of people to know. Everybody feels sorry for you and I don't want a lot of people to feel sorry for me.

FRIEND: I know you didn't want a lot of people to know. But Wanda had a miscarriage, too. I thought that she could be a good supportive person to you.

PROTAGONIST: I thought that I could trust you. I feel really let down.

DIRECTOR: Reverse roles.

"FRIEND" (P): *(Almost crying.)* I'm sorry. I am so, so sorry. I really thought I was doing something that would be helpful for you. Please forgive me.

DIRECTOR: Reverse roles.

PROTAGONIST: *(Stands there looking at the auxiliary friend, shaking her head in puzzlement. She says nothing and looks defeated.)*

DIRECTOR: I want to give you a double. *(A group member volunteers.)*

DOUBLE: *(Standing to the side and a little behind the protagonist.)* I am hurt by what you did but I am also angry with you for doing it.

PROTAGONIST: That's right! I am angry. I am really pissed off at you! How dare you break my confidence and then tell me you are doing it for my own good?

Soliloquy is also employed when the protagonist is in a role reversal with a significant other. Here the purpose is to assist the protagonist deepen the protagonist's understanding of the role of the significant other by attempting to delve into the subjective thoughts and feelings that the significant other might be experiencing in the situation. This is one of the tactics for the process that Moreno called social investigation.

Role Reversal

Several writers (Carlson-Sabelli, 1989; Marineau, 1989, for example) have pointed out that the psychodramatic technique of role reversal was foreshadowed in an early publication, *Ein Ladung zu Einer Begegnung* (J. L. Moreno, 1914), translated by Moreno as *An Invitation to an Encounter.* The passage, in English, is:

> A meeting of two: eye to eye, face to face.
> And when you are near I will tear your eyes out
> and place them instead of mine,
> and you will tear my eyes out

and replace them with yours,
then I will look at you with your eyes
and you will look at me with mine.

(1946b)

Role reversal is probably the most utilized of the basic psychodramatic techniques. It is very likely the most valuable as well. There are several situations in which a role reversal is called for. An absent significant other appears in almost every psychodrama. The term, significant other, applies to people, pets, and anybody that is germane to the drama. In most psychodrama situations, a member of the group is assigned to take the role, to be the auxiliary. In some psychotherapy groups, experienced staff members are used to take these auxiliary roles but a common practice is to ask the protagonist to choose the group member to play the absent significant other. Upon introduction of a significant other into the drama, directors usually ask the protagonist to reverse roles and become this person. Protagonists then present their perceptions of how the new individual looks, moves, thinks, and feels in the situation to be dramatized. This gives the director and the group members a sense of this other person and instructs the auxiliary on how to act when taking that role. Protagonists can simply describe their perception of the significant other, but getting the information through the action of role reversal is quicker, more comprehensive and efficient. The protagonist is then asked to assume his/her own role while the auxiliary takes the role of the significant other and the drama proceeds. An example:

DIRECTOR: So you are in your living room for this call. Where do you see your mother?

PROTAGONIST: Oh, she is probably on the porch. She has a large screened in porch at the rear of the house. It is like another room.

DIRECTOR: Let's use this part of the stage for mother's porch. *(Protagonist sets the scene.)* Who would you like to play the role of mother? *(Protagonist selects a group member to play the role.)* Reverse roles with mother. *(Gives protagonist a moment to do so.)* What is your name, mother?

MOTHER (P): Rosa.

DIRECTOR: Describe yourself for us, if you will. How tall are you? *(Continues to ask questions and the protagonist answers as mother. Then he asks:)* And how do you feel about your daughter?

MOTHER (P): Well, I am disappointed in her. I don't like her being gay.

DIRECTOR: I see. I'm sorry to hear that. Reverse roles. *(Auxiliary ego takes role of Rosa and protagonist resumes her role as daughter.)* Who makes the call, you or mother?

PROTAGONIST: I do. I call every Sunday morning.

DIRECTOR: Show us. *(Protagonist replays the phone call.)*

Role reversals occur throughout most psychodramas. They serve several purposes. After the protagonist has presented a significant other through role reversal, an auxiliary can often engage with and respond to the protagonist in ways that keep the drama proceeding. However, if the auxiliary injects something into the drama that is too disparate from how the protagonist perceives the significant other, the protagonist may object and momentarily lose his or her warm up to the psychodrama role. Role reversal in this instance provides a means to correct the auxiliary and return to the protagonist's warm up. An example:

FATHER (AE): Well, if you really feel that way about it, go ahead and do it.
PROTAGONIST *(TO DIRECTOR)*: He wouldn't ever say anything like that.
DIRECTOR: Reverse roles and show what he would say.
FATHER (P): Well, I guess I can't stop you if you want to fuck up your life that way. *(Shakes head in disgust.)*
DIRECTOR: O.K. Reverse roles. *(To auxiliary ego)* Play the role that way.

A role reversal is called for when the protagonist asks the significant other a factual question and the auxiliary cannot be expected to know the answer. The protagonist is reenacting a scene in which her relationship with her boyfriend was very positive. It is Sunday morning and they are having breakfast. The auxiliary ego has been portraying the boyfriend quite adequately without role reversals. The protagonist then asks a question and director knows that the auxiliary ego has no way of knowing how to respond:

PROTAGONIST: What are we going to do today?
DIRECTOR: Reverse roles.
BOYFRIEND (P): I promised Fred that I would help him move this afternoon. Then tonight we're going to a party at Robert's place.

Another important moment that calls for a role reversal is when a protagonist has confronted the significant other with an ethical question, a question that asks, in effect, "How do you justify your actions?" There are many variations ("How could you do that?" "Why did you do that?") and sometimes it is an accusation ("You lied to me!" "You cheated me!") It is associated with intense emotions of anger and hurt and possibly other feelings, often suppressed. After the protagonist has charged the significant other with such behavior, the director asks for a role reversal, often asking the protagonist in the role of the significant other to justify his or her actions with respect to the protagonist.

Perhaps the most valuable aspect of role reversal is that it allows protagonists to get a sense of what it is like to be the significant other and to experience a situation from the perspective of the significant other. It permits protagonists to get an idea of how the important people in their lives experience themselves.

Finally, and perhaps most importantly, it allows protagonists to view themselves through the eyes of significant others, to discover how they are experienced by the significant other. Zerka Moreno tells about the time when she first reversed roles with her young son, Jonathan. Warming up to the role of a little boy, Zerka watched Jonathan becoming his own mother. He stretched himself to his fullest height, tipped his head back and looked down his nose at "himself," being played by Zerka. It was the way a royal personage might look at a commoner. "My God!" Zerka thought to herself. "Is that the way my son sees me?"

There is another occasion in psychodrama when an immediate role reversal is called for and it is a rare occurrence. Protagonists have an amazing ability to respond convincingly to auxiliaries as the significant others whom they portray and, at the same time to be aware that they are actually stand-ins for those individuals. This serves to protect auxiliaries who are playing the roles of significant others with whom the protagonist is intensely angry. Protagonists almost never hit or strike or hurt an auxiliary. It is difficult to get most protagonists to hit an auxiliary with an encounter bat even though the bat, made of sponge rubber, is made for the purpose of hitting without causing damage. If a protagonist expresses a desire to hit or kick or otherwise do physical injury to the significant other, a variety of ways are used to protect the auxiliary. The auxiliary, maybe with help from another group member, hold a mattress or heavy cushions that the protagonist may strike or kick. The protagonist may express anger by striking a chair or box with an encounter bat. On very rare occasions, however, a protagonist in an over-heated state may actually inflict a physical blow on an auxiliary ego. The director should immediately call for a role reversal and instruct the auxiliary to return the blow exactly as they experienced it. Example: *The protagonist has expressed deep hatred toward his mother whom he perceives as having been a tyrant most of his life. He and the auxiliary mother are sitting face to face in an encounter. Suddenly, without warning the protagonist slaps the auxiliary across the face.*

DIRECTOR: *(Immediately)* Reverse roles! *(After protagonist and auxiliary have traded places the director says to the auxiliary now in the protagonist's role)* Slap your mother again, just as hard as you did before. *(As the auxiliary pulls back her arm, the protagonist in the role of mother puts up a hand to protect himself. Director instructs)* No! Don't put up your hand. *(Auxiliary in the role of the protagonist delivers a strong slap to the "mother's" face.)*

This immediate remedial action serves several purposes. Auxiliaries usually feel taken advantage of and betrayed on the rare occasions that this happens. The role reversal tends to even the score. The auxiliary knows that the protagonist has received a message by experiencing what he served. Most protagonists realize immediately that they have violated the auxiliary and tend to feel guilty and apologetic. Receiving the blow that he or she delivered can resolve the guilt, and allow the drama to proceed without further ado. In thousands of psychodramas in which I have participated, often as an auxiliary, I have seen a protagonist misuse an auxiliary in this way only a few times, and have been abused myself as an auxiliary only once.

Directors often invite the protagonist to reverse roles with objects as well as with people. Objects that we own and especially those we value highly are extensions of ourselves. Reversing roles with them often gives us new insights about ourselves and our values and always reveal subtle aspects of the protagonist to the group. These role reversals can help understand the protagonist and the situation at hand:

The protagonist is setting the scene of her room when she was about eleven years old. She indicates the size of the room, describes the bed and other furniture, using simple props like a mattress for the bed, chairs and a small table for other furniture.

DIRECTOR: Is there something in this room that is especially meaningful to you?

PROTAGONIST: Yes. Over here on this shelf is a tiny china doll that my grandmother gave me. It was hers when she was a child.

DIRECTOR: Would you reverse roles with that doll? *(The protagonist strikes a pose.)* I understand that you used to belong to Alice's grandmother but now you are Alice's.

DOLL (P): That's right.

DIRECTOR: And you mean a lot to Alice.

DOLL (P): Yes. She knew that her grandmother loved me very much so she knew that her grandmother must love her very much to give me to her. This family needs all the love it can get.

DIRECTOR: The family needs love?

DOLL (P): They do a lot of fighting and fussing at each other.

DIRECTOR: Is Alice happy? Does she have many friends?

DOLL (P): She is friendly but her family moves around a lot so she has trouble keeping friends. They have moved almost every year recently. *(The director keeps interviewing the doll and learns even more about the protagonist's situation during this time in her life.)*

It is often easier for protagonists to reveal important information in role reversal with either significant others or with objects than it is in their own roles. Pets, cats and dogs especially, often can tell us things about protagonists that the protagonists don't think to reveal about themselves. Another informative maneuver is role reversal with the spirit of a house or a room. This entity is then asked questions such as "What does the family that lives in you feel like?" "Is it a happy family, a close family?" "What do you see happening in you?"

Moreno writes that the role reversal is more effective the closer the two individuals are in psychological, social, and ethnic proximity. He considers it an advantageous learning device that helps correct unsocial behavior. Role reversal increases one's role perception and sociometric status. A person's skill in reversing roles is proportional to the number of roles that individual takes in life (J. L. Moreno, 1964).

Encounter

The concept of encounter is the fundamental principle of social interaction in Morenean theory and will be discussed in Chapter 5 on theory. With respect to psychodramatic action, two different processes are included in the term: the psychodramatic encounter; and the encounter *in situ*. A psychodramatic encounter occurs in practically every psychodrama. It is an encounter between the protagonist and a significant other, often involving a confrontation, with the significant other played by an auxiliary ego. The psychodramatic encounter often begins with the protagonist reenacting a scene in which the protagonist and significant other have had a misunderstanding or an argument. Sometimes it starts with the protagonist expressing outrage and anger at the significant, other accusing them of wrongdoing. The task of the director is to get a clear statement from the protagonist about what the significant other did that bothered the protagonist. The next step is for the protagonist to ask the ethical question: How do you justify or explain your actions? As soon as the ethical question is clearly stated by the protagonist, the director calls for a role reversal. This puts the protagonist in the position of justifying the significant other's behavior. The director then uses a variety of techniques to help the protagonist explore the subjectivity of the significant other such as interview, soliloquy, and doubling. In the role of the significant other, the protagonist may be defensive or even issue a counter charge, or possibly acknowledge that the accusation is valid. Regardless, a number of role reversals are apt to take place as the protagonist attempts to resolve the problem.

The *in situ* encounter is a directed encounter between two group members. The parties to the encounter might be a husband and wife, boyfriend and girlfriend, or supervisor and employee, who wish to explore their relationship. These are usually co-protagonist psychodramas and consist of reenactment of past events from the perspective of both people. The other situation that calls for *in situ* encounter is dissension between group members that they cannot or do not resolve between themselves. A group member may ask for an encounter because of uncomfortable feelings with another member of the group. The director or the group participants also may ask two members to have an encounter because negative feelings between them are affecting the group's well-being.

It is unlikely that there is anybody who can love everybody that he or she is thrown together with over the course of life. In almost every group to which we belong, work, church, social organization, hobby group, etc., there is somebody or some persons involved whom we wish were not. Sociometric research confirms that rejection is universal; almost everybody rejects someone, and almost everybody is rejected by someone. These negative feelings affect not only the individuals themselves but others in the group. A directed encounter between two people who have a strong dislike for each other is not likely to end up in their becoming great friends. An encounter can, however, result in a greater understanding of each other, and can reduce the negativity between them to the point that they can work together. Dealing with the conflict openly reduces its negative effects upon the group as well.

Directing an *in situ* encounter is a demanding task requiring a high degree of objectivity and neutrality on the part of the director. It is of utmost importance that both parties to an encounter feel that they have had an equal chance to express themselves. Usually the encounter begins with the co-protagonists facing each other. If one of these has asked for the encounter, the director will ask him or her to tell the other why. The other is then asked to respond. The feelings that each party experiences in relation to the other are critically important and the director uses soliloquy and doubles, if necessary, to make sure that these emotions are adequately expressed. At some point, a role reversal can assess how well the co-protagonists have heard each other. This should not be done early in the encounter. When a person has strong negative feelings towards another, it is difficult to reverse roles with that person. Instead of a valid role reversal, there is a tendency to produce a caricature of the other. This, of course, is not helpful to reducing tensions. It is also essential when directing an *in situ* role reversal that each individual is given a chance to correct what the other produces. Thus the director, as a way of concluding the encounter, may ask for a role reversal. A takes the role of B; B takes the role of A.

DIRECTOR: A, tell B how you are feeling toward him now, after your encounter.

PROTAGONIST A (PROT. B): *(Does so.)*

DIRECTOR: B, tell A how you are feeling toward him.

PROTAGONIST B (PROT. A): *(Does so.)*

DIRECTOR: Reverse back into yourselves. A, is there anything you want to correct or add to how B presented you? (*Allows A to respond.*) B, is there anything you want to correct or add to how A presented you? *(Allows B to respond.)*

It is very helpful to identify transference phenomena during an encounter. Either party may recognize that the other reminds them of a problematic relationship from past experience. This can lead to the psychodramatization of past events in the life of one or both co-protagonists. Replacement of transference with tele, that is, perceiving the other accurately and not through the filter of an earlier relationship, can be a powerful factor in improving the relationship between two people.

The Double

The most demanding task for an auxiliary is taking the role of the double. Rather than portraying a significant other, the double assumes the role of the protagonist. Assigned the role of the double, the double takes a position to one side of and slightly behind the protagonist and reproduces as far as possible the posture of the protagonist. In this location, the double is close to the protagonist and can watch out of the corner of the eye the protagonist's posture and movements in order to mimic them. At the same time, the double is largely out of the protagonist's sight.

Directors use doubles in several ways. The basic task of the double is to tune into the protagonist's inner feelings and thoughts and give voice to that which the protagonist is unable to articulate. In highly charged moments, we often are assailed by a number of emotions, each with its demand for expression, often conflicting with each other. For example, someone we love has acted in a way that we perceive as betrayal. Anger, pain, fear, and desire may all be competing and resulting in an emotional knot that we cannot untie. It is hard to identify what we feel and often we fight against expressing any feeling to avoid the uncomfortable emotions. The double's task is to help us identify, untangle, acknowledge and express all these feelings in the proper order. An example of this use of doubling is given in one of the scenarios in the section on role reversal above.

Although this may sound close to mind reading, it is not only possible but learnable, and some individuals have been trained by their life experiences to tune in quickly and deeply to the emotions of others. Although we think of emotions as personal and subjective, and learn many ways of concealing what we are feeling, there are many clues to the emotions that one is experiencing. Darwin (1872) first called attention to the role of facial expression and saw similarities between man and other animals. Paul Ekman (1999), a psychologist whose career has been devoted to the study of emotions, has confirmed that individuals from widely diverse cultures can read each other's facial expressions. Posture, gesture, and body movement also provide clues to one's feelings. and Moreno explored this phenomenon as reported in *Who Shall Survive?* (1953), this accounts for the instructions to the double to mime the protagonist. Certain qualities of voice, timbre, tonality, loudness, pitch, for example, are additional indicators of the emotion that one is feeling.

There is another process that I don't think has been adequately reported in the psychodrama literature by which we react to the emotions of another person. When we are in proximity to another person, we tend to respond to the emotional state of the other with similar feelings. In teaching doubling skills, I often use the analogy of two pianos in the same space. Striking a note on one of them causes the corresponding strings in the other to vibrate, a well-known phenomenon. When we are in proximity to another person, we respond to the emotional state of the other in a similar way. Interacting with someone who is highly anxious, we often become tense ourselves. Sitting and engaging with someone who is depressed may result in our feeling inexplicably tired or drowsy. Likewise, we often feel more positive in the presence of a confident or serene person. Like two pianos, we reverberate to our companions. This is a function of tele, a Morenean concept of unconscious communication that I will discuss in a later chapter on psychodramatic theory. The double, then, as a helper to the protagonist and assistant of the director, brackets and puts aside his or her feelings in order to tune into the emotions of the protagonist. Putting aside feelings like this is not something people ordinarily do spontaneously, but it can be learned.

During the early years of the development of psychodrama at Beacon Hill Sanitarium, Moreno trained nurses and other staff members to serve as auxiliary egos. Working with psychotic patients required an experienced auxiliary and an experienced auxiliary was of substantial help to the psychodramatic director-therapist. When Zerka Moreno, then Zerka Toeman, joined the Beacon Hill Sanitarium staff in 1942, she became Moreno's most frequently used auxiliary and she devoted herself to becoming the best auxiliary ego possible. She has published two articles dealing with her experiences, especially her work with psychotic patients (Toeman, 1946; Z. T. Moreno, 1978). Those of us who have experienced her skill to tune in and give voice to elusive feelings and thoughts are convinced that she achieved her goal of becoming the best auxiliary ever. Doubles have been used very creatively by psychodrama directors. Everybody has the experience of carrying on an internal dialog, of talking to oneself. The director can externalize subjective, internal conversation by having the protagonist talk to the double. I often say, "This is yourself. What do you want to say to yourself about this?" Conflicting roles or emotions can be represented by using two or more doubles, each representing a position in the conflict.

The Mirror

In order for protagonists to observe their own behavior, their posture, gestures, facial expression, tone and timbre of voice and the like, a director may ask protagonists to pick an auxiliary to be themselves, a double actually. The director takes the protagonist just off stage and asks the auxiliaries to re-play the last scene. The auxiliary chosen to take the protagonist's role is instructed to play the part exactly as the protagonist did. This is called the mirror and is intended to give protagonists an opportunity to observe themselves from the outside.

The mirror was often used at the Beacon Hill Sanitarium for oppositional and withdrawn patients who would not voluntarily go up on the stage as protagonist. Moreno would have a staff member who knew the patient's history act out scenes from the patient's life while the patient watched from the audience. The auxiliary had been cued to make a mistake during the portrayal of the patient. When this happened, the patient would often object. "That's wrong! That's not the way it happened!" Then the director would say, "Why don't you come up here and show us how it happened?" Patients usually complied, warmed up to action by seeing themselves mirrored by somebody else.

The mirror is also called into use to acquaint protagonists with body language and facial expressions of which they are unaware. An example: in a psychodrama, a young protagonist was exploring difficulties that had developed in her relationship with a lover. He had informed her that he felt smothered in the relationship and asked her for some distance. She had agreed to "give him more space." In role reversal, as the lover, she physically moved away slightly from the auxiliary who was now in her role. Reversed back into her own role, the auxiliary repeated the movement. She then took a step closer. The auxiliary took another step away. Again the protagonist followed and soon the two of them were moving around the stage, talking all the time, the lover trying to take a step away and the protagonist promising to give it to him but moving toward him. The director employed the mirror technique. He replaced her with a double and asked them to replay the last few minutes of enactment. As the protagonist watched, she asked in wonderment and some embarrassment, "Was I really doing that?" A more involved and complex use of the mirror is described in the chapter on directing a psychodrama.

The Empty Chair

Also called the four legged auxiliary by Moreno, the empty chair is used in lieu of an auxiliary ego. Protagonists are asked to picture the person to whom they wished to speak in a chair on the psychodrama stage. After confronting or otherwise engaging with the significant other, the director asks the protagonist to reverse roles and become the individual in the empty chair. By using the empty chair, the protagonist's spontaneity is not challenged by the counter spontaneity of an auxiliary. This can be an advantage especially for highly anxious protagonists. An encounter can start out with an empty chair and then be replaced by an auxiliary after the protagonist is more fully warmed up.

The empty chair figures in a classical group warm up exercise. The director invites group members to identify someone with whom they have unfinished business. Unfinished business is defined as something you need to say to someone but have never taken an opportunity to express. Unfinished business can be something connected with negative feelings toward the significant other or just the opposite, positive feelings that have not been articulated. Each member of the group is given a chance to make a statement to whomever they see in the empty chair and then to role reverse and reply.

An empty chair encounter and unfinished business can also be a way to demonstrate the psychodrama method to a new group. A volunteer is asked to picture someone with whom he or she has unfinished business in the empty chair (Warner, 1970). The first statement and the reply to it illustrate both self presentation and role reversal. An auxiliary can then be introduced and the encounter expanded, offering the possibility of introducing soliloquy, doubling, and possibly the mirror or the matryoshka doll techniques.

The empty chair was adopted by Fritz Perls and became a major element of his gestalt therapy, so much so that it was widely believed that Perls had originated it. Perls, influenced by his earlier training in psychoanalysis, rejected the interpersonal theory of Moreno, maintaining that one's behavior could be understood from within the individual. For him the auxiliary and the auxiliary's counter spontaneity contaminated rather than enhanced the process. Perls used the empty chair to deal with intrapersonal rather than interpersonal issues.

The empty chair achieved a certain notoriety during the 2012 presidential election in the United States. Actor Clint Eastwood presented half an encounter with President Obama at the Republican National Convention using an empty chair. Talking to the president, he criticized Obama's policies and actions according to Republican doctrine. However, as Jonathan Moreno (2012) noted in a *New York Times* op-ed piece, Eastwood failed to complete the encounter by reversing roles.

Occasionally, a protagonist presents a scene in which he or she has been abused in such an unconscionable way that the group members cannot find any understanding of the abuser's actions or state of mind. The sexual rape or extreme physical abuse of a young child are examples of these situations. In order to give the group a way to express the indignation and anger that the group experiences, the director can put an empty chair on the stage at the end of the action session to represent the perpetrator, inviting the group members to express their feelings toward him or her (Speros, 1972).

Director's Confrontation

Moreno claimed that it was permissible for the director to laugh or joke with protagonists as well as to challenge, confront or even shock them. This must be done without being hostile or aggressive. Here is an example:

The protagonist is reenacting a childhood scene. She is outdoors in the yard with three of her brothers, close in age. She would like to play with them but they gang up on and reject her. She is sitting under a large tree reading and the brothers are horsing around with each other near her. One has climbed up in the tree.

DIRECTOR: And what happens now?
PROTAGONIST: A pebble hits me on my head.

DIRECTOR: Show us.

PROTAGONIST: OW! That hurt! Cut that out!

DIRECTOR: Reverse roles.

BROTHER IN TREE (P): Sorry, it was an accident.

DIRECTOR: Reverse roles.

PROTAGONIST: (*Sighs and continues reading*) Well, O.K. Just be careful, will you? That really hurt.

DIRECTOR: Is that all you do?

PROTAGONIST: Yeah. (*Director looks at her questioningly.*) Well, he said it was an accident.

DIRECTOR: An accident! How the hell do you think that pebble got up in that tree? Was it by accident? (*Group members laugh. Protagonist looks taken aback.*)

PROTAGONIST: Oh. Do you think he did it on purpose?

DIRECTOR: Well, I've never seen rocks just setting around on tree branches waiting to fall off.

PROTAGONIST: Oh. I never thought of that.

A variation of confronting the protagonist in the protagonist's own role is the confrontation of a significant other and occurs when the protagonist has reversed roles with that individual. This is a technique that Zerka Moreno (n.d.) frequently used and one that I have adopted also. This is especially effective when a protagonist has accepted a significant other's claim for special privilege or for a position that the director thinks is unfair or unethical. An example:

A graduate student has been unable to finish his dissertation, all he needs to complete his doctorate. In an encounter with his grandfather, the grandfather, an immigrant who lost a successful business in the depression, cautions him about going out into the world. "The world will defeat you," is the message.

DIRECTOR: (*To the protagonist in the role of grandfather.*) Do you love your grandson?

GRANDFATHER (P): I love him very much.

DIRECTOR: Then why do you encourage him not to try? Why do you set him up to fail?

GRANDFATHER (P): I don't want to see him get hurt. I tried and thought I was doing very well. Then the depression came and wiped me out. I don't want him to get hurt like that.

DIRECTOR: He is a very bright young man who has every chance of succeeding. You are making him fail. Is that what you want to do?

The director's confrontation of the significant other is especially helpful when there is a disparity in status between protagonist and significant other so that it is particularly difficult for the protagonist to confront the significant other. The confrontation accomplishes at least two goals. It encourages the protagonist to experience the role of the significant other at a deeper level in order to account for that person's motivations. It also broadens the protagonist's perception of the situation by looking at from the perspective of the significant other. Additionally, the protagonist experiences the director as an ally, standing up for him or her, confronting the significant other in a way that the protagonist has been unable to do, speaking for the protagonist in a situation in which it is difficult for protagonists to speak up for themselves. It gives protagonists courage when they assume their own roles.

The director can also use this technique to counsel the protagonist in a very direct manner:

The protagonist wants to leave her husband who is overbearing and controlling, and with whom she has been fighting and arguing constantly. She cannot bring herself to make the break because of the objections of her five year old son who does not want the family to break up. She believes she needs to get his consent in order to leave. In a role reversal, the director talks to the son.

DIRECTOR: Kevin, you want your mom and daddy to stay together. That is only natural. Of course you want them both. But there are some things that you cannot fully understand when you are only five years old. Mom and dad fight a lot and mommy is getting depressed. She also thinks that it is not good for you to grow up in a house where there is so much tension. The only reason that she has not left is because you don't want her to go. But she may have to use her grown up understanding and wisdom and leave anyway. You won't like it and may get very angry with her. She may have to leave anyway and hope that one day when you are older and wiser, you will understand why she did it.

KEVIN (P): *(Nods as if he understands.)*

DIRECTOR: Reverse roles and let's finish up with Kevin and send him out to play.

Protagonists, it would appear, can more readily accept very direct messages from a therapist when delivered to a significant other, when they are in the role of that person. Perspectives and judgments that would otherwise elicit defensive rejection receive more careful consideration when presented this way. This is very direct approach, more so than many psychotherapists and psychodrama directors would ordinarily adopt, and should be used only when the director is quite comfortable with it.

Concretization

Although almost everything psychodramatic, and psychodrama itself, is a sort of concretization, or making tangible the subjectivity of a protagonist, this term is usually reserved for the enactment of a figure of speech. The technique is helpful for identifying the concrete figures and events behind the protagonist's metaphors and vague statements. Thus:

The protagonist has been selected without having identified a specific theme or issue that she wishes to explore.

DIRECTOR: What is it that we are going to explore in this psychodrama?
PROTAGONIST: Gosh, I'm not sure. There is so much going on in my life.
DIRECTOR: What are you feeling right now?
PROTAGONIST: (*Pauses to think.*) Well, I have a picture in my mind.
DIRECTOR: What is it?
PROTAGONIST: It is a car that's stuck in the mud and a tow truck.
DIRECTOR: O.K. Let's put that into action. Show us this car stuck in the mud and a tow truck. Set the scene. Where are we?
PROTAGONIST: We are out in the country. There is a road here. Over there it is woods. The car has run off the road and gotten stuck in the mud.
DIRECTOR: Reverse roles with the car.

After the protagonist has played the car and the tow truck, it is clear that she identifies with the car stuck in the mud. She now identifies a number of factors in her life that she sees as keeping her from moving ahead. The tow truck is a cry for help.

Protagonist's make many statements in the course of a psychodrama that can be concretized. Responsibilities are often described as bearing down on one or experienced as weight. The director asks the protagonist to pick an auxiliary to be themselves (a double) and then the protagonist becomes the weight. The protagonist then demonstrates how the weight is experienced. The roles are reversed and the auxiliary has been instructed on how to take the role of the weight.

Protagonists also feel responsibilities or other people pulling on them, pushing them, picking at them, restricting or restraining them, all of which can be put into action. Concretization can be very effective in giving the protagonist something tangible to deal with in the place of the intangible, subjective feeling with which they begin. The flexibility of psychodrama allows for the concretization every metaphor or simile.

Spontaneous Improvisation

This is a technique that Moreno used frequently but which is not much employed by psychodramatists today. Moreno's first attempt to treat a specific situation, the marriage of Barbara and George, began with improvisational drama as she was assigned the role of a prostitute in a Living Newspaper drama. Moreno continued using improvisation after he began to develop psychodrama systematically. He introduced several improvisational procedures at the Hudson Training School including the spontaneity test, the role-playing test, the situation test, and spontaneity training (see J. L. Moreno & Jennings, 1937). The technique involves the protagonist acting out fictitious roles and events rather than acting out experiences from the protagonist's own life. The situations involve conflict and a demand for action. For example, the subject is assigned the role of an employee who is being fired for coming in to work late, or a boyfriend who is accused of being unfaithful by his girlfriend. Sometimes an auxiliary is not required. For instance, the subject is in his home when he smells smoke and discovers a fire has broken out in one part of the house. He is informed that there is an infant in one bedroom and important papers in another part of the house, and someone is approaching the house to enter near the location of the fire. Whether it is a role test or a spontaneity test depends upon what the administrator of the test is investigating. When the situation is to explore the subject's ability to mobilize sufficient spontaneity in playing out imaginary or lifelike situations, it is a spontaneity test. When the purpose is to assess the range of roles and adequacy in playing them, it is role testing. Situation testing could guide further training for life skills. All served as spontaneity training. (J. L. Moreno, 1953b).

Moreno used these instruments extensively in his reconstruction of the Hudson Training School society. He also illustrated their use in marital therapy in *Psychodrama, First Volume* (1946b). He reports working with a couple, Robert and Mary. Robert has a serious anxiety disorder and it is complicated by marital problems. Moreno assigns them a series of role relationships, such as sheriff and shoplifter and district attorney interrogating a suspect criminal, that they are instructed to enact on the stage. The purpose is partially diagnostic and partially to increase their spontaneity in relation to each other. Improvisation allows an individual to experience psychodramatic roles, roles that they would like to play in life but cannot for various reasons, including social pressures or lack of opportunity. Today, improvisation is utilized less frequently by psychodramatists. Improvisational theater training, however, makes extensive use of such exercises.

Matryoshka Doll Technique

This is a technique that I began using after reading an article by Robbins on children's warm up exercises for adults (M. Robbins, 1973). Among the many exercises described here was one called the matryoshka, referring to the Russian nest of dolls, traditionally decorated as the grandmother. My variation is a social investigation technique, designed to better understand the feelings and thoughts of a significant other. I use it when a protagonist is puzzled by a significant other's behavior and cannot account for it in simple role reversal with the significant other. It is easier to illustrate than explain, so here is an example:

PROTAGONIST: (*Whose mother is in a nursing home with degenerative brain disease, is angry at her brother who won't go visit her. Through role reversal, the protagonist has shown how the brother responds to her demands that he visit.*) If you would just go once in a while, it would help. She keeps asking about you.

BROTHER (AE): Look, I am taking care of the finances for her. That's enough. I just don't have time to go visit. You see her a couple of times a week but you have the time to do it.

PROTAGONIST: Yes, you are doing the financial thing and God knows I am so thankful for that. I love you for that. But—Go and visit her!

BROTHER (AE): (Raising voice) I don't have the time.

DIRECTOR: Reverse roles. (*To the protagonist in role reversal*) What do you feel when your sister begs you to go visit your mother?

BROTHER (P): Irritated. I'm angry. I do my part, she does her part. Why can't she leave it at that?

DIRECTOR: Pick someone to be angry brother. (*Protagonist does so.*) Now put a chair a little behind and to one side, and sit in it. (*To angry brother auxiliary*) Repeat your line, angry brother.

ANGRY BROTHER (AE): (*To protagonist*) I am angry with you. I do my part. You do your part. Let it go at that!

DIRECTOR: (*To protagonist*) Sit there until you have another feeling, another emotion.

PROTAGONIST: (*After a pause*) Yeah, I feel sad.

DIRECTOR: Soliloquize.

PROTAGONIST AS SAD BROTHER: I am sad. I know that Mother is losing her mind. It is a sad situation.

DIRECTOR: Pick someone to be sad brother. (Protagonist does so.) Put another chair behind and to the side. (*Has auxiliary for sad brother speak the lines.*) Sit there until another feeling comes to you.

PROTAGONIST: (*Another pause.*) I am scared. I'm scared she's going to die. (*Tears come into protagonist's eyes.*) I feel terribly afraid. (*At this point, protagonist drops out of role and speaks as herself.*) I didn't know my brother felt so afraid. He's always seemed so confident and strong.

DIRECTOR: New thought, huh? Let's try another one. (*Protagonist continues the exercise and experiences several more feelings. Director then reverses her back into herself and asks her to continue the confrontation with her brother, speaking to any one of the "brothers" or to them all as one.*)

This technique makes use of the fact that in any situation we inevitably have a number of emotional responses to a corresponding number of emotional stimuli. These emotions vary in strength, in how aware we are of each, and in how willing we are to express each. We tend to be most aware see and react only to the most obvious one, the one on the outside. These emotions are identified and separated by this technique just as the series of dolls are disclosed as we open a matryoshka doll. It is important that the protagonist follow the instruction to sit quietly in the next chair until a different emotion is detected. Protagonists are often skeptical when asked to "sit there until another feeling comes to you," but it invariably does, and the protagonist feels the emotional change clearly and strongly. The director who is tuned into the protagonist may be aware of the feeling that the protagonist will identify before the protagonist says it. The number of emotions that the protagonist can identify varies greatly. Six or seven are not unusual and I directed one protagonist used eleven chairs in her drama. Eventually, the protagonist will report experiencing no new feeling.

Other Techniques

This discussion is not intended to serve as an exhaustive explication of psychodramatic techniques. It is, rather, a brief survey of the most commonly used psychodramatic devices and especially those that I tend to call upon as a psychodrama director. A search of the psychodramatic literature will reveal a number of others. Many articles discuss the techniques used with particular populations. For example, for training police in family crisis intervention (Barocas, 1972), resolving racial tension in the schools (Ferinden, 1970), and students with Asperger syndrome (Munir, Scholwinski & Lasser, 2006). New techniques are invented whenever a psychodrama director discovers a unique way to help a protagonist express an internal thought, feeling, memory, or conflict in action.

References

Barocas, H. (1972). Psychodrama techniques in training police in family crisis intervention. *Group Psychotherapy & Psychodrama*, 25, 30–31.

Carlson-Sabelli, L. (1989). Role reversal: A concept analysis and reinterpretation of the literature. *Journal of Group Psychotherapy, Psychodrama & Sociometry*, 41, 139–152.

Darwin, C. (1872). *The Expression of the Emotions in Man and Animals*. London: John Murray.

Ekman, P. (1999). Basic emotions. In T. Galgleish & M. Power (Eds.). *Handbook of Cognition and Emotion*. Hoboken, NJ: John Wiley & Sons. 45–60.

Ferinden, W. E. (1970). Multidimensional approach in resolving racial tension in the schools utilizing psychodramatic techniques. *Group Psychotherapy and Psychodrama*, 91–96.

Hudgens, M. K. (2002). *Experiential Treatment for PTSD: The Therapeutic Spiral Model*. New York: Springer.

Karp, M. (1998). The director: Cognition in action. In M. Karp, P. Holmes & K. Bradshaw-Tauvon (Eds.). *Handbook of Psychodrama*. London: Routledge. 129–146.

Marineau, R. (1989). *Jacob Levy Moreno, 1889–1974*. New York: Routledge.

Moreno, J. D. (2012, September 1). What the chair could have told Clint. *New York Times*, A23.

Moreno, J. L. (1914). *Ein Ladung Zu Einer Begegung*. Vienna: Anzengruber Verlag.

Moreno, J. L. (1937). Inter-personal therapy and the psychopathology of inter-personal relations. *Sociometry*, 1, 9–76.

Moreno, J. L. (1940). Psychodramatic treatment of marriage problems. *Sociometry*, 3, 1–23.
Moreno, J. L. (1944). A case of paranoia treated through psychodrama. *Sociometry*, 7, 312–327.
Moreno, J. L. (1946a). Psychodrama and group psychotherapy. *Sociometry*, 9, 249–253.
Moreno, J. L. (1946b). *Psychodrama, First Volume*. Beacon, NY: Beacon House.
Moreno, J. L. (1953). *Who Shall Survive?* Beacon, NY: Beacon House.
Moreno, J. L. (1958). Fundamental rules and techniques of psychodrama. In J. H. Masserman & J. L. Moreno. (Eds.). *Progress in Psychotherapy Volume III: Techniques of Psychotherapy*. New York: Grune and Stratton. 86–131.
Moreno, J. L. (1959). Psychodrama of Adolf Hitler. In J. L. Moreno in collaboration with Z. T. Moreno, *Psychodrama, Second Volume*. Beacon, NY: Beacon House.191–200.
Moreno, J. L. (1964). The third psychiatric revolution and the scope of psychodrama. *Group Psychotherapy*, 149–171.
Moreno, J. L. & Jennings, H. (1937). Spontaneity training, a method of personality development. *Sociometric Review*, 17–25.
Moreno, Z. T. (1978). The function of the auxiliary ego in psychodrama with special reference to psychotic patients. *Group Psychotherapy, Psychodrama & Sociometry*, 31, 163–166.
Moreno, Z. T. (1965). Psychodramatic rules, techniques and adjunctive methods. *Group Psychotherapy*, 18, 73–86.
Moreno, Z. T. (n.d.) Psychodrama in action. www.psychotherapy.net/video/Psychodrama-in-Action-Zerka-Moreno, accessed June 28, 2014.
Munir, S., Scholwinski, E. & Lasser, J. (2006). The use of psychodrama techniques for students with Asperger syndrome. *Journal of School Counseling*, 4, 2.
Nolte, J. (2008). Protagonist without a problem. In J. Nolte (Eds.). *The Psychodrama Papers*, Lulu.com, 173-174.
Robbins, M. K. (1973). Psychodramatic children's warm-ups for adults. *Group Psychotherapy & Psychodrama*, 26, 67–71.
Speros, T. (1972). The final empty chair. *Group Psychotherapy & Psychodrama*, 25, 32–33.
Toeman, Z. (1946). Clinical psychodrama: Auxiliary ego, double, and mirror techniques. *Sociometry*, 9, 178–183. (Reprinted with commentary in T. Horvatin & E. Schreiber (Eds.) (2006), *The Quintessential Zerka)*.
Warner, G. D. (1970). The didactic auxiliary chair. *Group Psychotherapy*, 23, 31–34.

3

WARMING UP

The *warming up process* is an integral component of Moreno's concept of spontaneity–creativity, the theoretical foundation of all his contributions. Warming up is defined by Moreno as the operational expression of spontaneity. All creative acts at all levels of creativity, physical, biological, and human begin with warming up. Warming up is preparation for action and plays a role not only in psychodrama but also in every creative act from the emergence of a new star, to the appearance of a new species, to every act we perform, every action we take. David Kipper (1967) pointed out that among psychodramatists, there has been confusion of the concept of the warming up process with spontaneity, as well as confusion between the concepts of the warming up process and the warming up phase of a psychodrama session. This chapter deals with the warming up phase, the first part of a psychodrama session that leads to the selection of a protagonist for the action phase. The more theoretical warming up process is discussed in Chapter 7 of this book.

The Warming Up Phase

The warming up phase of a psychodrama session begins with the gathering of the members of a group and continues until a protagonist has been selected. At that time, the action phase of the session or drama proper begins. Students of psychodrama quickly learn the importance of the warming up process to the successful conduct of a psychodrama session. An appropriately warmed up group functions more smoothly in many ways, the selection of protagonists and directors, the warming up of the protagonist, and the flow of the drama itself. A properly warmed up group feels satisfied at the conclusion that the proper protagonist has been selected and that the session has successfully achieved its goal.

There are actually many warming up processes to a psychodrama session and they all play an important part in what happens in the session. First, every participant to an upcoming psychodrama session or psychodrama training workshop warms up to the event in his or her own way. This takes place wherever the person happens to be and may occur place partly in the participant's awareness and possibly outside it. Whenever an individual thinks in advance about an upcoming psychodramatic event, she or he is warming up to that occasion. The warming up may be positive or negative. One group member may eagerly anticipate the event. Another may experience anxiety every time she or he thinks about it. A third may look forward to seeing other group members while another warms up to negative feelings about one or another of the participants. Warming up processes of group members will likely include thoughts about what might happen during the session, desires to be a protagonist or director, fears of being protagonist or director, and countless other emotions. These thoughts and feelings tend to grow stronger and more frequent as the moment for the session approaches. The initial task of the group is identifying these various currents of emotion to which its members are warming up, and discovering how to proceed to the maximum fulfillment for the whole group. That is the objective of the warming up phase of a psychodrama session.

The group leader warms up as does every other group member, experiencing anxiety perhaps or anticipation or both. Factors that will influence the group leader/director's warming up include the nature of the group, whether it is a psychodramatic therapy group in an inpatient setting, an outpatient group, a substance abuse group, a personal growth and development group, a psychodrama training workshop, a role training group for doctors, nurses, lawyers, or department store managers, an organizational development event, a public demonstration of psychodrama, or one of a myriad of other possibilities. Obvious factors for the leader to consider include the extent to which membership in the group is voluntary, the ages of the group members, the number of sessions that this specific group has had or will have, whether the group is an open group or a closed one. A particularly important element is how the various members feel about being in the group, whether they prefer to be or want not to be in the group. A subtle factor that influences the group is the sociometry of the group, the reactions of group members to each other and how these feelings play out in the group's functioning. Many elements play a part in the warming up of the group to psychodramatic action and these dynamic processes in flux can generate anxiety in even an experienced group leader.

The goal of the warming up phase is to get the group started:

> In all forms of extemporaneous psychodrama the chief problem is how to get the group started. The best prescription is to let the warm up come from the group itself. Anything can start the ball rolling. There is

> no one who begins and there is no favorite topic. It may start with a joke, with an outburst of anger of one member of the group towards another or towards someone not present ... Experience has shown that what appears to be a planless beginning gradually leads to a significant process of production, as if it would have been carefully planned. In the course of such actions, abreactions, interactions, interabreactions, role playings, dialogues, interviews, discussions, analyses, one or another individual or a clique of individuals comes forth with a special problem. It comes spontaneously to an acting out unless the atmosphere is purposely restricted and unless there is a silent consensus that action are taboo. Otherwise, acting out will take place within the group itself and thus the action portion of a psychodrama session begins ... The use of acting out techniques makes the responsibility of the director greater and requires a special skill of direction, but their inclusion has therapeutic and research advantages.
>
> *(J. L. Moreno, 1953a, pp. 73–74)*

In this passage, Moreno describes a maximally unstructured warming up phase. In one of the earlier articles on psychodrama and group warm up, Enneis (1951) writes that warming up

> is a process by which the group focuses. By the merging of varied interests, it centers on a problem area with which it is willing to be concerned during a particular session. There is an exclusion of peripheral concerns, and a crystallization of the more basic areas with which the group will deal.
>
> *(p. 17)*

Enneis (1951) and Yablonsky and Enneis (1956) elaborate on this approach to warming up in a psychodrama group. They describe two common patterns that occur when a group leader remains passive during the warming up phase, and one in which the leader plays an active role.

The Cluster Warm Up

In the warming up strategy that Yablonsky and Enneis call the *cluster* warm up, the director remains passive as the group gathers and starts talking among themselves. Several small clusters spontaneously form around different topics. Eventually, a cluster moves to a topic that draws the attention of the other small groups. As the little groups cluster together, other group members who have not been involved become engaged and a topic of concern to all is recognized. The protagonist, the individual in whom the problem area seems most clearly crystallized, is identified and the psychodrama begins.

The Chain-of-Association Warm Up

The *chain-of-association* warming up process tends to occur in a group in high spirits, Yablonsky and Enneis write. As they come into the room, laughing and making playful remarks off each other, someone says something that draws the whole group into a serious mood and discussion. The theme of the group soon evolves. The group member who seems to best symbolize the problem is selected as protagonist and the drama moves into action.

Directed Warm Ups

Enneis and Yablonsky also discuss *directed* warm ups. The *leader directed* warm up is often used in training groups when a particular theme or issue needs to be explored. The leader identifies the issue, warms the group up to it, perhaps by discussing the need for the group to experience and investigate it. The drama that follows is limited to that issue. Another form of the directed warm is *group member* directed. A group member who wants to explore a personal problem may warm the group up to her or himself by announcing the desire to be the protagonist, perhaps giving a brief statement of the issue to be considered. On occasion, the group itself will direct the warm up to a member whom they wish, for one reason or another, to be the protagonist, a *group directed* warm up.

Warm Up Exercises

In a discussion of the warming up process, Moreno (1953b, pp. 337–340) introduced the notion of *starters,* instigators of the warming up process. He discusses several types of starters, physical, mental, interpersonal, and social. A *physical starter* consists of a set of movements which tend to activate a specific feeling. For example, a protagonist who cannot mobilize the feeling or expression of anger is directed to clench teeth and fist, stare and frown and walk heavily around the stage. *Mental starters* are directions to the protagonist to warm up to expression of a specific emotion or state. A simple example of *interpersonal starters* is the direction to "visualize someone to whom you have something to say in the empty chair. Then say what you have to say." *Social starters* in the form of short exercises in which group members interact in a structured way have become very common in the psychodrama collective and are generally referred to as warm ups. An example: the group members sit in a circle and the instruction is for each member in turn to say a single sentence. The group leader may start the exercise with a theme such as "Make a sentence about how I feel at this moment." Additional subjects can be introduced: "Something I like about myself;" "Something I dislike about myself;" "How I feel toward by parents;" and the like (Weiner & Sacks, 1969). *All starters have the goal in common of instigating or increasing an emotional state which intensifies the tendency to act.*

When I was training at the Moreno Institute during the 1960s, there was intense interest in warm ups, a recognition of the importance of the warming up process in the practice of psychodrama. Many of my fellow trainees were quite energetic in collecting and exchanging warm ups with each other, as was I. Dozens of these exercises, many of them coming from encounter groups of the Human Potential Movement, have been generated and traded back and forth. Carl Hollander, who was a fellow student of the author at the Moreno Institute, gathered and marketed a collection of 100 warm ups as *The Warm-Up Box* (Hollander & Hollander, 1978). Literature on warm up exercises includes: Pramann (1990); Sacks (1967); and Weiner and Sacks (1969).

These social starters can be effective expedients in moving a group into action even though they are in conflict with Moreno's principle of letting the warm up come from the group itself. The structured exercise reduces the anxiety that many people feel at the beginning of session, especially in a newly formed group. Appropriately designed for the specific situation, a warm up can increase group cohesion and activate the emotions that will eventually lead to the psychodrama itself. Warm ups can be even more effective in reducing the anxiety of the psychodrama director, especially the novice director.

Warm ups, however, can be overused. There is a growing practice among psychodrama directors and trainers who have been trained in the last several decades to begin every session with a structured warm up exercise. This may reflect inadequate comprehension of the concept of the warming up process as well as a confusion of warm ups with the warming up phase. The warming up phase begins as group members, each with their own personal warming up to the session, come into the space in which the session takes place. At this point, the telic and transference relationships (see chapter on theory) begin to influence the warming up of the individual members of the group before any warming up exercise is introduced. The experienced director looks for ways of facilitating expression of these factors in the group. Other well-known psychodramatists, including Marcia Karp and Anne Ancelin Schützenberger (Karp, 1998) and William Wysong (2017), join me in disparaging the practice of injecting a warm up exercise into every psychodrama session.

Few groups need a structured warm up exercise after the first session or two. Unless designed specifically to identify or alleviate interpersonal issues that are inhibiting the group's work, a warm up exercise can interfere with the natural flow of a cohesive group and delay rather than facilitate its process into psychodramatic action. It thus accomplishes the opposite of the goal of the warming up process. The most effective psychodrama directors are those who trust and rely upon their own spontaneity to guide the warming up process of the group rather than those who randomly pick an exercise from *The Warm Up Box*. The warming up phase of a psychodrama session ends with the selection of a protagonist.

Selection of the Protagonist

There are several ways in which a member of the group becomes the protagonist. Moreno preferred the spontaneous emergence of a protagonist from a non-directed warming up process as described by himself and by Moreno and Enneis as discussed earlier. The least spontaneous procedure is the selection of the protagonist by the group leader or director. In between is a method that has become a part of the warming up phase of many, perhaps most, currently active psychodramatists. It is based on sociometric principles and is especially appropriate for group-centered sessions.

Personal growth and development groups and psychodrama training groups are typically group-centered, meaning that the social dynamics of the group are given the highest consideration in how the group functions. In small groups of six to nine members, there is often a consensus upon who is to be the protagonist in the current session. The protagonist is a high value role, however, and in larger groups there is often competition for the role. A widespread convention is to use a sociometric procedure for protagonist selection when more than one member is under consideration. In the sociometric choice process, members of the group who have expressed a desire to be the protagonist for that session are invited to make known the problem, issue, theme, or experience which they wish to explore psychodramatically. Each individual gives a brief statement, "I want to deal with a problem I have with my husband, (wife, boss, son, daughter, friend, etc.)" or "I have been feeling very down, very low energy lately, and I can't figure out why." Sometimes prospective protagonists are asked to reveal the issue by putting it into a newspaper headline, "Died and Brought Back to Life," a movie title, "Sad and Lonely," or in some other novel way. When the several issues are clearly communicated, group members are asked to ascertain which theme is most important to them personally. They indicate their choice by joining the protagonist who has proposed it. In groups where more than one individual is capable of directing a psychodrama, and two or more potential protagonists are heavily chosen, a large group can be subdivided into several smaller ones, each of which can conduct a drama. This is most common in psychodrama training groups. Where the situation does not allow for more than one drama, the individual with the most choices usually becomes the protagonist.

Not all groups are conducted in a group-centered manner, and the sociometric method is not always the best way of selecting the protagonist. In psychiatric settings where the purpose of the psychodrama is psychotherapy, the group leader may have reasons for choosing a particular member of the group to be the protagonist. The reasons are many. A member of the group has been avoiding the role of protagonist. Another member is too frequently chosen if the group is given responsibility for making the choice. The needs of one or another group member are for some reason of high priority. In these cases, the director must know how to warm up a specific group member to becoming the protagonist and simultaneously how to warm the group up to that group member. Martin Haskell, an early graduate of the Psychodrama Institute, demonstrated a subtle and easy way to warm any member of the group up to the role of protagonist at the 1963 Annual Conference of the American Society for Psychodrama and Group Psychotherapy. In a group of about 75 people, he asked a committee of 3 volunteers to choose any member of the group for the demonstration. Their choice was identified to Haskell only.

Haskell invited some volunteers to the stage, and asked them to select a current civic issue, take sides and debate it. He brought several people into the debate and dismissing others. Within a few minutes he said to a person (who had not been one of the first volunteers) "would you like to explore why you feel that way in a psychodrama?" The person addressed replied, "Well, yes. I would." Haskell looked toward the committee who confirmed that this was the person that they had selected.

References

Enneis, J. (1951). The dynamics of group and action processes in therapy: An analysis of the warm-up in psychodrama. *Group Psychotherapy*, 4, 17–22.

Hollander, C. & Hollander, S. (1978). *The Warm-Up Box*. Denver, CO: Psychodrama Center.

Karp, M. (1998). The director: Cognition in action. In M. Karp, P. Holmes & K. Bradshaw-Tauvon (Eds.). *Handbook of Psychodrama*. London: Routledge. 129–146.

Kipper, D. (1967). Spontaneity and the warming up process in a new light. *Group Psychotherapy*, 20, 62–73.

Moreno, J. L. (1953a). Preludes of the sociometric movement. In J. L. Moreno (Ed.). *Who Shall Survive?* Beacon, NY: Beacon House. 13–108.

Moreno, J. L. (1953b). *Who Shall Survive?* Beacon, NY: Beacon House.

Pramann, R. (1990). Warm Ups: For Your Back Pocket. www.ssccc.com/articles.htm. Accessed February 4, 2015.

Sacks, J. M. (1967). Psychodrama: The warm up. *Group Psychotherapy*, 20, 118–122.

Weiner, H. & Sacks, J. (1969). Warm-up and sum-up. *Group Psychotherapy*, 22, 85–102.

Wysong, W. (2017). *The Psychodrama Companion*. Lulu.com.

Yablonsky, L. & Enneis, J. (1956). Psychodrama theory and practice. In F. Fromm-Reichman & J. L. Moreno (Eds.). *Progress in Psychotherapy, Vol. 1*. New York: Grune & Stratton. 149–161.

4

CREATING THE DRAMA

The basic psychodrama techniques are relatively easy for a student director to learn. Co-creating a classical, protagonist-centered psychodrama, on the other hand, requires proficiency in a complex set of skills which is far more difficult to master.

> As producer [the director] has to be on the alert to turn every clue which the subject offers into dramatic action, to make the line of production one with the life line of the subject, and never to let the production lose rapport with the audience.
>
> *(J. L. Moreno, 1946a, p. 251)*

This is the set of skills that are so important and require a huge investment of time, training, and experience to learn. A director often faces many choice points in a psychodrama, choices of when to suggest a new scene or continue with the current one, choices of which of the clues a protagonist offers will be most productive, and choices with respect to the techniques that can best help protagonists express their inner thoughts and desires.

To make matters even trickier, these skills are frequently diametrically opposed to the skills in which one has been trained as a psychotherapist. The psychodrama director actively, sometimes forcefully, instructs the protagonist to reverse roles, soliloquize, or express feelings in action. This is a substantial contrast to the calm, reflective psychotherapist, listening closely, asking thoughtful questions and occasionally commenting on or interpreting the narrative of the client. Mastering the art of the psychodrama director has a long learning curve that accounts for the extended training period required for certification in the method.[1]

Warming the Protagonist up to Action

The choice of protagonist has been made. The group warming up process transitions into the action phase, the psychodrama proper. The group members take their places around the periphery of the stage. Now the director and protagonist must warm up to their respective roles. The experienced director may take a moment to reflect upon any of his or her own personal tensions that might intrude into the role or any feelings toward the protagonist that need to be acknowledged and put aside or "bracketed," in order to direct from a position of openness and neutrality. The novice director often needs to deal with the anxiety of being in an unfamiliar role. The first task of the director is to warm the protagonist up to the protagonist role, the issue to be explored, and to the spontaneity state. The director guides the protagonist into action.

The Initial Interview

Warming the protagonist up to action commonly begins with the initial interview, a topic discussed in Chapter 2. The director asks the questions he or she needs in order to clarify the problem or situation that the protagonist wishes to explore. As I pointed out in Chapter 2, the initial interview has several goals, the most pressing of which is to find a way to begin the drama, to identify the first scene. Moreno's (1954) recommendation was to learn just enough to get the drama into motion. He warned against letting the protagonist tell the story: "Don't tell us; *show* us!" has since become a psychodrama catchphrase. A common problem that novice directors have, especially those who are experienced psychotherapists when they come to psychodrama, is conducting an excessively long interview. This is due in part to the fact that interview is the primary modality of most forms of psychotherapy and the psychotherapy trained student director is more comfortable with interviewing than with directing action. Inexperience and anxiety also may prevent neophyte directors from perceiving clues that the protagonist provides to possible first scenes. The first scene is important because it serves to warm the protagonist up not only to the theme but also to action instead of narration. Moreover, the first scene acts to warm up the audience to the protagonist as they see her or him interacting with the significant others in her or his life. Creating the first scene further deepens the relationship between the director and the protagonist.

A short initial interview gets the protagonist into action as quickly as possible. Action helps reduce whatever anxieties the protagonist may have. Action also engages the group members to a greater extent than does interview. Finally, it also obeys the psychodramatic preference for showing what happened over talking about what happened.

A number of psychodramatists who have been trained in recent years have been taught a more extended version of the initial interview called the *walk and talk*, and this has become a standard procedure for many directors, which, in my opinion, is unfortunate. The protagonist is directed to walk the periphery of the stage with the director, perhaps holding hands. The protagonist is encouraged to describe various aspects of his or her issue or story in an effort to discover the focus of the drama. The protagonist and director, according to Garcia (n.d.), decide where the drama will take place. They may plan the first scene or agree to several scenes. She writes:

> The walk and talk is also the time when the director and the protagonist contract for the scope and goals of the work. The director will ask such questions as, "What do you want to happen in this drama?" or "What will let you know that this drama has succeeded?" or "What do you want to happen by the end of the drama?" or "What do you want to be sure to do in the enactment?" or "What do you want to come away with from this drama?"...
>
> By the end of the walk and talk, the director and protagonist know the following: where the action will take place; what characters will be in the drama; and what the contract is. The director may also have a working hypothesis of what issues the protagonist is dealing with and how he may help him in the drama
>
> *(Garcia, n.d.)*

In short, the director and protagonist have essentially planned the psychodrama. Planning ahead may very well reduce the director's anxieties, but it tends to create an outline for the drama in advance. Expectations of what is going to happen can limit the psychodrama by discouraging the director from following up on unanticipated clues that develop during the action. The plan attenuates the spontaneity of both protagonist and director as well. A psychodrama should be a spontaneous exploration of the protagonist's inner subjectivity. Neither the director nor the protagonist need know ahead of time where the psychodrama will lead. As Moreno (1953a) wrote,

> The more prepared and planned the production is, therefore, the more a psychodramatic session resembles a production in the legitimate theater. The potential participants of the audience behave more and more like spectators; they are passive and receptive ... Do not pay the price of spontaneity for smoothness, regularity, orderliness, continuity and elegance.
>
> *(pp. 75–76)*

Dramas are far more effective when directors trust their skill and the spontaneity of the protagonist and let the story unfold in action. The protagonist's warm up is reduced by talking about the event in advance of the drama. The audience's warm up is similarly lessened by knowing in advance what will happen. "The less of the story of the incident is given to the audience in advance, the more involved will be the protagonist and the more spontaneous his production will appear to the audience" (J. L. Moreno, 1954, p. 165). Planning can limit choices that might lead to critical scenes for the protagonist's self understanding. Many powerful dramas deal with events that are beyond the possibility of the protagonist or the director to know before the drama begins. Once scenes, characters, and outcomes are announced in advance, they serve as guideposts and can inhibit introduction of other elements into the drama. In my opinion, a preferable procedure is to get the drama started and let it unfold from the first scene.

The First Scene

Every event occurs in a specific place and at a specific time. This is true even of fantasies and dreams. Life consists of situations and an important aspect of every situation is the place where something happens. The psychodrama stage provides a flexible medium that can become any place on earth, in outer space, in fantasy, in heaven or hell. The formal stage constructed especially for psychodrama is not necessary but does facilitate the production of psychodrama. In most groups, the stage is a designated area of a room around which group members sit in a circle or semicircle.

Scene setting is an important technique that enhances the warming up process of the protagonist, transforming the empty stage space into a place that has meaning for the protagonist. This is especially true when the locus of the psychodramatic scene has great significance for the protagonist. Important events such as encounters often take place in kitchens and bedrooms. Recreating the room with simple props and ample description aids in making reenactment feel real for both protagonist and audience.

Finding a starting point, establishing the first scene is actually not particularly difficult. It can be brought forth simply by asking the protagonist to recall an experience that illustrates the issue that he or she wishes to explore. Another approach recognizes that the drama is a story from the protagonist's life. The protagonist is asked, "Where does this story begin?" On occasions when the protagonist cannot state the issue or problem clearly or identify an experience associated with it, the director can ask that the protagonist warm up to the emotions stirred up by the issue. Moreno called this a "mental starter" (J. L. Moreno, 1953b, p. 340). When the protagonist has warmed up to the emotion, the director asks the protagonist to identify the situation or location in which the emotion is most strongly felt. The protagonist's response becomes a potential first scene. An effective first scene is an action statement of the problem that the protagonist has presented. For example:

The protagonist is a professional man about 37 years old attending a weekend psychodrama training workshop. The problem he would like to explore has to do with abandonment by a girlfriend with whom he had lived for two years. "I feel lonely a lot and I miss her," he states. The director knows that the protagonist has explored the break-up with Trisha in a previous psychodrama. Otherwise, he might have suggested beginning with the scene of the breaking up or with the protagonist's first hint of a problem in the relationship. He reminds the protagonist of the earlier psychodrama and at the same time fills in other group members who had not been present at it:

DIRECTOR: We have explored the break up with Trisha recently in another drama, haven't we? So it seems to me we need to deal with the lonely feeling that seems to be keeping you from moving on. Does that make sense to you?

PROTAGONIST: Yeah. My sister wants to set me up with someone she knows and I just can't seem to get interested in going out with someone new.

DIRECTOR: When do you have this lonely feeling the most strongly?

PROTAGONIST: When I am at home.

DIRECTOR: When was the last time that you felt it and it was really strong?

PROTAGONIST: (*Without hesitation.*) Last night. I took my dog to my parent's house to stay while I am at this workshop. It was when I came home I really felt lonely.

DIRECTOR: And where in your house were you when you were aware of how lonely you felt?

PROTAGONIST: In the kitchen. I had just come in.

DIRECTOR: Take us there. Set the scene.

The protagonist has done a number of psychodramas previously and spontaneously begins to describe the kitchen. The director asks questions to elicit details that help the protagonist and the group to imagine the scene. The initial interview has taken less than one minute before the protagonist is into psychodramatic action. After the scene is set, the protagonist will show us the situation in which he feels lonely and is missing his relationship with Trisha.

Unfolding the Drama

Every psychodrama is a unique event. No two people have the same exact experience even though they may be involved in the same event—even twins. At the same time, it is exceedingly rare that we can't all relate to the event in one way or another. Commonality of experience is the factor that makes sharing possible and ensures that a psychodrama session is relevant to all members of the group. We learn over and over that no matter how different we are from each other, and certainly we are each one-of-a-kind, we are all still more alike than we are different. However, the infinite variety of situations that protagonists present for exploration makes serious demands upon the director to be both spontaneous and creative.

Many, perhaps most, psychodramas deal with protagonists and their problematic relationships with members of their social atoms. Dissension between spouses, family conflicts, disputes with neighbors, co-workers, fellow members of organizations, a difficult supervisor, and other sources of discord are familiar instances. The protagonist is directed through scenes that illustrate the problem. Protagonists reverse roles with the significant others to look at the situation, and themselves, through the eyes of significant others to achieve expanded understanding of the situation. In the freedom and safety of the psychodrama stage, and with the use of role reversal, doubling, and other techniques, protagonists obtain new and broadened perceptions of the situation, of significant others, and often of themselves. The director may then assist the protagonist to experiment with creative ways of resolving the friction or controversy that exists. An example:

In a role training workshop for medical resident physicians, an eye surgery resident was exploring his anger and frustration with a patient, a young Black woman whom he was seeing without a fee in a special clinic set up for impoverished people. He reenacted the scene in which he had seen her. He made a careful and professional examination of the eye, told her she had an infection, and treated it. His demeanor was quite professional and proper. In role reversal, he presented her as sullen and even dismissive of him. He wondered if she realized how serious her situation was. He told her how she needed to take care of the infection and gave her a prescription:

PROTAGONIST: It is very important that you use those drops three times a day. Let me show you how best to do it. Use your thumb and forefinger to open the lids like this *(shows her what he means by opening his own eyelid)* and squeeze out just one drop on the eye. *(Protagonist indicates he wants to do a role reversal.)*

DIRECTOR: Reverse roles.

PATIENT (P): *(Appears disinterested in what he is telling her, bored even. Gives a deep sigh.)*

DIRECTOR: Soliloquize.

PATIENT (P): Big fucking deal. I'm wasting my time here.

DIRECTOR: Reverse roles.

PROTAGONIST: *(Very seriously.)* It is really important that you take care of that eye just like I told you. If you don't you could lose sight in it.

DIRECTOR: That's what you said and I imagine that is the way you said it. What would you *really* like to say?

PROTAGONIST: (*Jumps up.*) GOD DAMN IT! YOU'D BETTER LISTEN TO ME INSTEAD OF SITTING THERE LIKE A KNOT ON A LOG. AND YOU'D BETTER DO WHAT I TELL YOU. (*Takes a deep breath. Talks to the director.*) That's what I felt like doing. I felt like she was going to ignore everything I told her and that she could easily lose that eye. I just wanted to shake her. Make her listen to me.

DIRECTOR: You sound to me like you were really concerned about her. Like a good doctor should be.

PROTAGONIST: Yes. I was—am—concerned about her. She looked to me like her life wasn't all that great and she certainly didn't need to lose that eye. I was pissed that she didn't seem to be listening to me.

DIRECTOR: Reverse roles with her. Show us Barbara's (*the name that the protagonist had given the patient*) posture. Walk like Barbara. Let's see Barbara's expression. Feel what it feels like to be Barbara. (*Pause to let protagonist reflect*). Okay, Barbara, tell us a little about yourself.

PATIENT (P): (*Drops out of role.*) I really don't know very much.

DIRECTOR: Feel yourself into the role as best you can. (*Gives him a moment.*) How old are you?

Since his knowledge of his patient is rather limited, it is more of a sociodramatic role reversal than a psychodramatic one. That is, the protagonist is playing the role of a young, impoverished Black woman more than the role of this particular young Black woman who was his patient. Finally the director asks:

DIRECTOR: Okay. Now tell me what are you feeling? How does it feel to be you?

PATIENT (P): Not real great. I feel pretty depressed. Sorta hopeless. Life is a drag. My eye bothers me a lot but it is just one more thing. Now I've got to spend some money for medicine and I don't have much as it is.

DIRECTOR: How do you feel toward the doctor who just saw you?

PATIENT (P): He's okay I guess.

DIRECTOR: He seemed pretty concerned about you.

PATIENT (P): I dunno. He probably doesn't give a fuck about me. He probably sees me as the infected eye. My eye is just one of my problems. My life is pretty bad right now. (*The young resident's posture is slumped. It looks like his feelings are congruent with the words he is putting in his patient's mouth. The director continues the interview a little longer.*)

DIRECTOR: Let's do one more thing. Let's let you have a talk with Barbara now that you've tried to see things from her point of view.

PROTAGONIST: I'm not angry at you now like I was. I tried to treat you like any other patient that I see. That was wrong. I should have treated you like you, like who you are, not like everyone else. I should have taken a little more trouble to find out who you are, why you seemed so disinterested in what I was trying to tell you. I took it as a personal insult. I think I have learned something in doing this. And I can say I was truly concerned about you and your infected eye.

Other psychodramas begin with a problem in the protagonist's current life but then end up dramatizing and exploring a painful or fearful event in the protagonist's childhood. Children have a number of such experiences as they acquire the rules and standards of family and social behavior. We frequently learn by inadvertently violating familial or cultural codes of behavior and as a result we are corrected, punished, and even abused. Some of these experiences are intense enough to have a residual impact on our lives. Other experiences that continue to affect us long after the fact come from failures in achieving our goals in interpersonal relationships and social situations. Rejection when attempting to establish a friendship or by a popular clique is extremely painful to school children, as is failure in the classroom or playground. Being teased, bullied, and made fun of are other examples of incidents that easily have effects that last long into adulthood. Time and again such experiences have a quality of unfairness or injustice. These incidents also have a characteristic of something unfinished or uncompleted. An example:

The protagonist is a Native American man in his 30s. A mental health professional, he has undergone psychotherapy and has considerable insight into his own functioning. He presents as the problem that he was abused by his grandmother when he was a small child and he thinks this continuing anger at her results in his becoming intensely angry at older women. He would like to confront his long dead grandmother in psychodrama in hopes of getting over this anger.

DIRECTOR: Before we encounter your grandma, I wonder if you could first show us a time when you got angry at an older woman. This way we can all see what it is that is a problem for you.

PROTAGONIST: O.K. Just this last week at work. I got angry with my supervisor.

The protagonist acts out getting a note that the supervisor wants to see him. He suspects that it is because he got into a heated argument with another staff member. He acts out the scene of the meeting with the supervisor. The supervisor likes and respects him but is often exasperated by his problems with other staff. He can be demanding and unbending at times. He in turn likes and is respectful to her and takes her admonitions appropriately. However, he must restrain intense anger to do so.

The director encourages him to express the anger and for the next ten or fifteen minutes, the protagonist does so. He screams and yells at her and tells her she is old and incapable of doing her job. She should quit. He punches a mattress held in front of the auxiliary supervisor. The director gives him a variety of ways to express the full intensity of the anger and encourages him to give full voice to it. Just when it seems that there is no end to it, the rage suddenly subsides and the protagonist begins sobbing. The director encourages him to lie on the floor. His body shakes with sobbing. The director encourages him to express his obvious pain with sound.

DIRECTOR: (*On the floor with the protagonist.*) Say "ow." (*Protagonist does so and sobbing intensifies.*) Grunt or groan. Push the pain out.

PROTAGONIST: Unhnhnh! Ohhhh. (*After some minutes, protagonist lies quietly. The sobbing and crying cease.*)

DIRECTOR: What are you thinking about, Paul? What do you see in your mind's eye?

PROTAGONIST: All the times I was abused.

DIRECTOR: Let's take a look. (*Both get up from the floor.*) What events are you thinking about?

PROTAGONIST: Being slapped in the face by my mother.

DIRECTOR: Place a chair to represent that time. (*Protagonist does so.*)

PROTAGONIST: And the time she hit me in the head with a soup can?

DIRECTOR: She hit you with a soup can?

PROTAGONIST: Yeah. I was acting up in the store.

DIRECTOR: Place another chair for the soup can. What else?

PROTAGONIST: Being strapped by teachers.

DIRECTOR: How many teachers strapped you?

PROTAGONIST: At least three that I can think of. (*Chairs are placed to represent these.*)

DIRECTOR: Go on.

PROTAGONIST: My Grandma, of course. (*Chair is added.*) And I almost got raped when I was in jail by these two guys. I was able to fight them off, though. I almost killed one. (*Pause.*)

DIRECTOR: Let's take a look at all these chairs we've put on the stage. The stage represents your life space. Looks like there has been an awful lot of abuse.

PROTAGONIST: (*Nods.*) Yeah. There has been. I hate this anger in me.

DIRECTOR: Yes. I think I understand. You don't want to pass it along by hurting others. What I am thinking, Paul, is that it would be helpful to you to revisit every one of these experiences psychodramatically. That's way too much for us to consider for one session but we can begin. Where would you like to start?

P: With Grandma.

DIRECTOR: She is no longer living, is she?

P: No.

DIRECTOR: You've seen enough psychodrama to know that we can invite her back by letting an auxiliary play her role. Whom would you like to invite to play that role? (*An auxiliary is picked and takes a seat on the stage facing the protagonist.*) What do you need to say to Grandma, Paul?

PROTAGONIST: Why did you do that? Why did you abuse me? I was only four years old.

DIRECTOR: Remind her what she did to you.

PROTAGONIST: You played with my genitals when you bathed me. I didn't know what to make of it. It made me uncomfortable. I didn't know what to make of it. And then you threatened to kill me if I told anybody. And you put me in the cellar. It was dark and there were snakes there and I was so scared. (*Protagonist begins crying.*)

DIRECTOR: It was black dark, wasn't it. And you were so scared.

PROTAGONIST: And that musty smell. I can smell it now. And I have so much anger in me. I have been violent. I hate that. I hate the violence in me.

DIRECTOR: Reverse roles. (*To "Grandma."*) How does it feel to hear that. To hear what your abuse of your little grandson has done to him?

GRANDMA (P): I feel ashamed. I feel disgust. I should not have done that to you.

DIRECTOR: What was your life like, Grandma? What happened to you?

GRANDMA (P): Oh, I was abused, too.

DIRECTOR: At least you are willing to acknowledge your abuse and your remorse. Would you do differently if you had it to do over again?

GRANDMA (P): If I could.

DIRECTOR: Reverse roles.

PROTAGONIST: I believe it. I really felt the disgust in her role.

DIRECTOR: Disgust with herself? With what she did?

PROTAGONIST: Yes.

(*The encounter continues and the protagonist expresses his anger at Grandma for how she abused not only him, but his mother, her daughter who then abused him in return. In role reversal, he elaborates his thoughts about how Grandma herself was abused as a child. Eventually the encounter is completed and Grandma allowed to return. The protagonist appears lost in reflection and the director waits for a few minutes until the protagonist looks up.*)

DIRECTOR: Let's go back to the scene in the supervisor's office.

The scene is recreated and the auxiliary repeats her lines, telling the protagonist to tend to his program and not get into fights with other staff members.

PROTAGONIST: (*To the director.*) I don't feel it. I don't feel the rage at her.

DIRECTOR: How do you feel about her?

PROTAGONIST: She is a good director. I know she likes me and is supportive of me. She thinks I do good work.

DIRECTOR: She just asked you to stick with your program and not tell others how they should run theirs? Respond to her.

PROTAGONIST: (*To supervisor.*) I understand. I know you are right and I will do better that way. *(And the drama ends.)*

Every emotion is a signal to the individual experiencing it to act in a specific way. The director in recognizing that the protagonist is angry at a significant other in the reenacted scene encourages the protagonist to express the anger that could not be expressed or expressed fully in the original event. Another feature of emotion is that when an emotion has been fully (or sufficiently) expressed, it subsides and a different emotion takes its place. A director needs to be very sensitive to this moment and to quickly identify the emerging feeling. Very often, after expressing intense anger and rage, a protagonist will feel hurt and pain and the director may need to facilitate the expression of that. On the other hand, the protagonist may feel a sense of calm or confidence after the expression of anger. This emotion, of course, is expressed in a very different way.

A frequent problem is the inability of protagonists to identify their own feelings, a situation that has been given the name alexithymia. There are several variations of the condition. Some people seem unable to recognize that they are feeling anything at all. More common are those who know that they are feeling something but cannot find a name for the emotion. This is the traditional time to call for a double to assist the protagonist. Another way to identify an emotion is to ask the protagonist what the feeling make him or her want to do. The answer is the key to the emotion. Wanting to run away means the feeling is fear. Wanting to beat, hit, kick, signals anger. Wanting to embrace is desire or love or a combination of both. Because most problematic situations, the kind that are explored on the psychodrama stage, involve a number of emotions, often conflicting ones, the director's task may be to help the protagonist sort out which emotion is the one that most needs to be expressed.

Some Psychodrama Conventions

Every experienced psychodramatist develops certain strategies for dealing with frequently encountered issues in the practice of psychodrama. In the discussion of psychodrama techniques in Chapter 2, I mentioned that some of these common courses of action are listed by authors as techniques but that I think of them as conventions, courses of action comprised of combinations of basic techniques. These protocols are conserves but not rigid rules. All of them allow for a maximum of spontaneity on the part of the director and the protagonist. A number of these practices were learned by students of the Moreno Institute when that training facility was in operation and have continued to exist, being passed down from trainers to trainees through several generations. Others have been developed over the years by other psychodrama directors. Here is a handful of them.

Childhood Abuse Scenes

In discovering the origins of irrational behaviors or reactions, the protagonist if often reminded of uncomfortable events from early in life. Scenes of childhood abuse are relatively common in psychodramatic work. There is a very wide range of actions on the part of parents that can feel abusive to children and that can have an unseemly or adverse effect upon their lives far into adulthood. On what the milder end of a continuum are undeserved criticism and punishment, and being teased or ridiculed. At the other extreme are such events as severe physical punishment involving tissue damage and/or sexual abuse.

Such experiences are associated with pain, fear, and anger, suppressed by the conditions of the situation in which they occurred. All of these emotions need to be expressed by the protagonist to neutralize the effects of the event. Most protagonists can be helped to access and express the pain and fear emotions. Anger can be more difficult to deal with. In the reenactment of scenes of abuse, the pain is often accessed in an intense abreaction. However, with protagonists strongly warmed up to their roles as children, the differential in power between child and parent makes it impossible for the protagonist to stand up to the father or mother, no matter how unfair or abusive that parent is being. The director is often confronted with an impasse. The protagonist is angry at the significant other while fear of incurring even greater abuse or of abandonment inhibits a satisfactory expression of the anger.

The mirror provides a solution for coping with the problem. Assume that the abuse scene has been produced. The protagonist's mother has accused her eight year old daughter of misbehavior and is punishing her. The protagonist in the role of her younger self is lying on a bed and is being beaten on her back and legs by the mother with electrical cords. The protagonist has demonstrated both roles and an auxiliary ego has taken the role of mother. The protagonist is loudly begging the mother to stop hurting her. The mother is loudly berating the daughter. The director stops the action.

DIRECTOR: Freeze! Stop the action! (*To the Protagonist.*) Pick somebody to be your eight year old self.

PROTAGONIST: (*Asks a group member to take the role.*)

DIRECTOR: (*To the Protagonist.*) Come out of that role. (*To Auxiliary.*) Take the role. Lie down on the bed. (*To the Protagonist.*) Stand here with me as your adult self. (*Both stand just off stage.*) (*To both Auxiliaries.*) Replay the scene. (*Auxiliaries do so. After a few minutes, to the Protagonist.*) As you watch this what does it make you want to do?

PROTAGONIST: Make her stop beating her!

DIRECTOR: Then do it! Go into the scene and make her stop.

PROTAGONIST: (*Enters the scene and restrains Mother Auxiliary.*) Stop it! Stop hitting her! She didn't do anything bad! She's a good little girl! (*The Director now directs an encounter between the Protagonist and Abuser.*)

In some dramas, the abuser will admit to being wrong. In others, the abuser will maintain that they have the right to do whatever they were doing. Which version occurs is dependent upon what the protagonist produces in role reversal. Either way, after the encounter, the abuser leaves the stage and the director asks the protagonist to respond to the abused child, explain why he or she was being abused. Many protagonists are very nurturing to the child-self, explaining that the treatment was unfair and not the child's fault. *It is important that a role reversal takes place so that the protagonist in the child role hears what the adult self has said.*

There are many variations of this procedure. The protagonist may choose to deal with the child first, rescuing him or her from the situation. It is important for the protagonist to then confront the abuser afterward.

If an abuser expresses regret, the director can produce a helpful reparative scene:

DIRECTOR: (*To Mother (P).*) Would you do something different if you had it all to do over again?

MOTHER (P): Yes. I would if I could.

DIRECTOR: We are going to give you an opportunity that life can't, a chance to do things differently. Let's go back to the start of that scene. (*The Protagonist in the role of Mother with an auxiliary playing her younger self replays the scene and changes Mother's behavior as she would like. Then the revised scene is played once more with Protagonist in role of her younger self and original auxiliary for Mother in that role.*)

If Mother (P) says that she would like to do something different but doesn't know how, the director can have the protagonist show her. The Auxiliary Mother is called in to watch while the protagonist shows her how to deal with the eight year old child.

Expressing Anger

Sometimes the protagonist in the role of the parent does not believe that the parent would be willing to behave differently, given the chance. Some people have the misfortune to be parented by or to encounter individuals who seem to them to have no redeeming virtue of any kind. Parents, and other adults, who sexually abuse children, and parents, grandparents, and others who physically abuse to the point of causing tissue damage often fall into this category. Seriously neglectful parents, sadistic bosses and supervisors and bullies qualify as well. Protagonists who bring psychological wounds from such a relationship to the psychodrama stage usually need to disencumber themselves of intense, perhaps murderous, anger. Protagonists will often have a specific action which they want to take. A protagonist may want to yell or scream at, hit, pound on, kick, stomp, or rip apart the offending significant other. The problem is to permit a full expression of rage without allowing protagonists to harm either auxiliary egos or themselves. The protagonist's awareness that the auxiliary is a stand-in for the actual person towards whom their rage is directed can inhibit the full expression of the feeling. Directors have devised many ways for protagonists to express their wrath at the those who have committed outrageous acts against them. Encounter bats and batakas are often used to physically express the anger, most often swung down upon the seat of a chair placed in front of the auxiliary significant other. This can make a very satisfying noise. To safely accommodate hitting, a mattress may be placed in front of the auxiliary, perhaps braced and held in place by additional group members. The mattress may be placed on the floor for the protagonist to stomp on and trample the offending abuser. A strong cardboard box can be given to the protagonist to rip apart. Large pieces torn off can be handed to the protagonist to reduce to smaller pieces for as long as necessary to fully express the protagonist's feelings. At the Moreno Institute, folding chairs were thrown against the back wall of the stage to the point where the wall had to be reinforced with a sheet of one inch thick plywood. That practice created a great deal of noise, which was very satisfying to protagonists who were so angry with an offending significant other that they were afraid of their own rage.

"Get Out of My Life!"

Many of us become engaged at some time with an individual who has a decidedly destructive influence upon our lives. There are some parents who are bereft of nurturing instincts, teachers who tyrannize and intimidate students, bosses and supervisors who do the same, and assorted and sundry bullies who occasionally enter into our lives and our life space. When it becomes clear a protagonist sees no way to achieve reconciliation with a significant other who has been excessively hurtful, or has no desire for any further contact with that individual, the protagonist may be invited to push the significant other out of his or her life. Example from a training group psychodrama:

The protagonist has completed a long and explosive expression of intense anger and hate toward the uncle who had repeatedly forced sex upon her during her preteen years, and had bullied her into not telling her parents. Reversed into his role, she can find no sense of regret or shame on his part. She has finished by ripping a sturdy cardboard carton into small shards. Finally she stops and looks at the director as if to say, "What now?"

DIRECTOR: Well, Gloria, it seems to me that you really don't need Uncle Karl in your life any longer.

PROTAGONIST: No. I haven't seen him in a long, long time and I don't ever want to see him again.

DIRECTOR: Perhaps you need to push him out of your life.

PROTAGONIST: I would like to do that.

DIRECTOR: O. K. Come here *(takes her to one edge of the stage area and calls the auxiliary playing Uncle Karl over.)* Here's how we will do that. The psychodrama stage represents your life space. *(The director arranges the protagonist and auxiliary so that they are facing each other at one end of the stage. Near the other end of the stage, the director designates a line.)*

Here is the boundary of your life space. I am going to let you push Uncle Karl out of your life for good. (The *auxiliary's back is toward the boundary line.)*

(To the protagonist) Put your hands on Uncle Karl's shoulders. Now push him out of your life, across that line down there. The rules are no biting, hitting, or kicking. Just push.

PROTAGONIST: *(She pushes the auxiliary fairly easily.)*

DIRECTOR: *(Stops the action.)* Reverse roles. Let's see how hard it is to get Uncle Karl to go. *(In Uncle Karl's role, the protagonist exerts far more resistance to being pushed out than the auxiliary had previously done. The director stops the action, reverses roles, and tells the auxiliary to use the same amount of energy that the protagonist had exerted.)* Now, let's try it again.

PROTAGONIST: *(Pushes auxiliary again. This time it is much harder.)*

DIRECTOR: Use your voice. Tell Uncle Karl to get out. Get out of your life!

PROTAGONIST: *(Pushing)* Get out! Get out of my life! *(They are approaching the boundary.)*

DIRECTOR: (*Stops the action.*) Freeze! (*To the protagonist*) Your throat is tight. Can you feel the tension in it? Loosen it up and lower your voice and say GET OUT OF MY LIFE! Go ahead. Push him out.

PROTAGONIST: GET OUT! GET OUT OF MY LIFE!

DIRECTOR: That's better. A lot better. (*Stops the action as Uncle Karl goes over the boundary line.*) How does that feel?

PROTAGONIST: (*Panting from exertion.*) It feels pretty good.

DIRECTOR: Then let's do it again. Come on back here.

The pushing out can be repeated any number of times depending upon the protagonist's desire to do it again. The director can tell when the protagonist has satisfied his or her need to push the significant other out. When the final push occurs:

DIRECTOR: Reverse roles. Well, Uncle Karl, how does it feel to be pushed out of Gloria's life?

"UNCLE KARL" (P): I didn't know she was so strong.

DIRECTOR: She is quite strong, strong enough that you cannot torture her again. But what I want to know is how does it feel to be pushed out of her life?

"UNCLE KARL" (P): *(looks puzzled and is thinking.)* I don't know. I haven't seen her in years. I don't think about her. *(Pause.)* She's the one who has been keeping me in her life.

DIRECTOR: Reverse roles. Say anything you want to finish with Uncle Karl.

PROTAGONIST: I guess he's right. I have been keeping him in my life. But I don't think I have to any more after this. *(She seems to be in deep reflection. To Uncle Karl in a determined voice)* And you stay out.

DIRECTOR: *(Lets the protagonist savor the moment for a while. When she seems to return from her thoughts)* I think it is time to share with our friends.

This scenario of symbolically pushing somebody out of one's life, someone whom the protagonist sees as no longer providing any benefit, serves several purposes. Even though it will physically tire the protagonist out, the pushing out exercise gives the protagonist an awareness of her or his own strength against a significant other who has previously felt overwhelmingly more powerful than the protagonist. This act also affirms for the protagonist that he or she is entitled to make decisions regarding those with whom to engage and with whom not to engage in life. Moreover, the exercise provides a feeling of satisfaction at the end of a psychodrama. Finally, it provides audience catharsis (see Chapter 7) for the group members who are emotionally experiencing anger at the injustice of the situation in which a significant other who has harmed the protagonist expresses no regret. This is no small matter because even though we refer to the event as the protagonist's psychodrama, it is actually a group production, "our" psychodrama. When we watch an individual being cruel to and exploiting another, the protagonist, we experience the tension of ethical anger. We want to see justice restored and the protagonist triumph. Pushing the bully out of the protagonist's life serves this goal.

Dream Psychodrama

Dreams have fascinated human beings forever. Dream interpretation, deciphering the strange reality of the dream world, has been an art if not a profession at least since biblical days when Joseph deciphered the dreams of the Egyptian Pharaoh. As happened in Egypt, dreams have often been considered portents of future events. Numerous books have been written to tell us what various dream symbols augur. Sigmund Freud took a different perspective, seeing dreams as the royal road to the unconscious, revealing unacceptable sexual urges rather than as omens of the future.

J. L. Moreno developed a procedure for dramatizing dreams that allows the dreamer to interpret the dream by putting it into action. The dream psychodrama gives individuals a chance to experience their dreams in a greater, more tangible reality, and in so-doing, to gain autonomy over dream patterns. The process is explained and demonstrated in several publications (J. L. Moreno, 1951, 1952, 1959, 1966).

Protagonists most often bring one of three kinds of dreams to the psychodrama stage. Nightmares that occur only once; repetitive nightmares; and dreams that seem unusually important to the dreamer but are puzzling at the same time. Moreno claimed that psychodramatizing a repetitive dream always ends it. My experience so far tends to confirm this.

Although psychodrama *always* calls for flexibility on the part of the director, the psychodrama of a dream ordinarily has five phases. The drama begins with anchoring it to the specific time and place that it occurred. The protagonist is directed through the actions of going to bed, undressing, washing, brushing teeth, etc. In bed, the director asks the protagonist to soliloquize the thoughts going through his or her mind as he or she falls asleep. The next step is to visualize the dream as it originally happened. The protagonist is asked to signal when the end of the dream has been reached. This may be by opening the eyes, maybe sitting up if the dream awakens the dreamer. Now the dream is dramatized. The usual procedures are followed with one major exception. Auxiliary egos are instructed not to expand upon the roles that they are assigned. The rationale is that in a dream, all the spontaneity comes from the dreamer, not from the other as in waking encounters. After the dream has been dramatized as it was experienced by the protagonist, the director offers an opportunity to redo the dream, making any changes that the protagonist would like to make. This is particularly helpful when the dream is a frightening one. Finally, the dreamer returns to bed and is instructed to have the reconstructed dream in place of the original one.

The following dream psychodrama took place during a workshop that was conducted in conjunction with a university class. The protagonist informed the group that she had a recurring nightmare. Even though it only happened about once a week, she had reduced the time she slept every night in an effort not to have the dream. She was willing to dramatize it. After the preliminary scene setting, that followed the procedure described above, in which the protagonist enacted going to bed and having the dream, she opened her eyes and sat up to indicate the end of the dream:

DIRECTOR: What is the opening scene of your dream?

PROTAGONIST: I'm in a car on a country road.

DIRECTOR: O.K. Let's set that up. *(Chairs are placed to represent the car. Protagonist sits in the driver's seat, holds on to steering wheel.)* What kind of car is this?

PROTAGONIST: A big black car.

DIRECTOR: Are you alone? How fast are you going?

PROTAGONIST: Yes, I'm alone. I'm going along pretty fast. I'm anxious to get there. It is night time.

DIRECTOR: Where are you going?

PROTAGONIST: Home, it is Christmas.

DIRECTOR: And what is happening?

PROTAGONIST: Now I am up to the fence, a white board fence. I can see the house over there. *(Points ahead of herself and to the left.)* I can see the lights, the Christmas tree lights. The kids are still up. I am driving along and I know that pretty soon I'll come to the gate. And I know that the gate will be open for me. They've left it open for me. *(She continues driving, then begins to look perplexed.)*

The director continues to direct the drama just as if it were an actual experience. As she nears where the gate should be, she can no longer control the car. It speeds up, the brakes don't work, and she can't steer. She becomes frightened.

DIRECTOR: Brakes don't work. Door won't open. What are you going to do?

PROTAGONIST: I'm helpless. I take my hands off the wheel. The car is driving itself. The house is receding. A hill is coming up. I am going to go up the hill. And when I go over the hill, I know that there will be nothing there. (*She becomes very upset.*)

DIRECTOR: O.K. Let's go up the hill now. (*Coaches auxiliary to tip her chair backwards.*)

Up the hill. (*Pause.*) Now we come to the top (*pause*) and now we go over. (Pauses a moment.) What is it like? Are you suspended in space? Are you falling?

PROTAGONIST: Don't know. I'm just there. I am suspended. I don't know what this place is. I don't know how I got here. I don't know why I'm here. (*Pause*) And now I start falling. (Screams) NO! NO! NO! NO! NO! NO! NO! I don't want to die!

DIRECTOR: Is there more?

PROTAGONIST: No. I wake up.

DIRECTOR: Soliloquize.

PROTAGONIST: *(awake)* Damn! Will that never stop? Will I ever get used to this?

So far in the psychodrama, the protagonist has dreamed the dream and has then put the dream into action. The next step is to extend or re-dream the dream. In some dreams, this is accomplished by letting the protagonist continue the dream past the point where it ended or woke the dreamer up. Other times this step is realized by asking the protagonist to change the dream in action. Both maneuvers are possible and the direction is taken depends upon the director's intuition or it may be negotiated with the protagonist. In this dream, the decision was to redo the dream.

DIRECTOR: (*to protagonist*) I'll tell you what we are going to do. We are going to let you have this dream all over again. Only this time, I want you to change it in any way and at any time that you want. How shall we begin?

PROTAGONIST: I like the way the dream starts. I am in a big black Lincoln that is full of presents and I am headed home.

DIRECTOR: O. K. Set it up. (*Protagonist does so and drives down the road.*) Let me know when you come to the fence. (*When protagonist indicates that she has come to the fence director asks group members to stand in a line to represent the fence.*) What happens now?

PROTAGONIST: (*As she drives along*) The gate is there and I turn in. (*The "Fence" makes a gap and protagonist turns in.*) And I drive up to the house. I can see the Christmas tree through the window.

The rest of the drama is a Christmas Eve party with the protagonist's children and her boyfriend. They sing carols and exchange gifts and finally the children go off to bed. The director clears the stage and auxiliaries go back to being group members.

The final phase of dream psychodrama is to have the protagonist dream the extended or modified drama. The scene is the initial scene in which the protagonist first reenacted having the dream.

DIRECTOR: Let's go back to the beginning of our drama. Set up your bedroom again. (*Protagonist does so.*) Get back in bed and go to sleep. (*Pause*) Now, dream your new dream. I don't think this one will wake you up. This psychodrama was reported in greater length in Nolte, Weistart and Wyatt (1977).

Future Projection

We are continually faced with making decisions about taking action and what actions to take. The majority of these we make easily or with only a minimum of effort. Occasionally we are confronted with major decisions that can have a life-changing impact upon our lives, decisions like getting married, having a baby, changing jobs or even careers, and the like. These issues require considerable and careful thinking through and can result in a high degree of uncertainty and anxiety. Some individuals have quite well formed and explicit goals toward which they are advancing. Every major decision is made with that objective in mind. For others, goals are less well defined and less often thought about. None the less, ambitions for the future, vague or precise, conscious or unconscious, influence how we act in the present.

One of the ways that psychodrama can be brought to bear on such issues is the future projection (Yablonsky, 1954). The director asks protagonists to pick a time in the future and put into action their ideas of where they might be, who will be in their lives, how they will be living, what they will be doing, etc. In addition to making protagonists conscious of strivings and internal forces of which they may be unaware, the future projection permits an exploration of the source of ambitions for the future. The protagonist is allowed to do this for every possible solution to the issue. The protagonist might project a future in which he or she took a new position as well as a future in which she or he stayed in the same position. An example:

A protagonist is very unhappy in her marriage; her husband is satisfied with it. They have seen a marriage counselor without much effect for her. However, she is quite fearful of leaving her husband, afraid of unbearable loneliness, of not finding another mate, and of being on her own. The director suggests that she project herself into the future.

DIRECTOR: Eve, let's look into the future. Imagine yourself five years from now. (*Pause*) Where do you see yourself?

PROTAGONIST: You mean if I stay married to Jim or if I leave?

DIRECTOR: It is your choice, and we can look at both. Which shall we do first?

PROTAGONIST: Five years from now? (*Long pause*) I have left. I left my marriage, oh, let's say four years ago. I am living in an apartment in Chicago.

DIRECTOR: So you have moved from Jacksonville. Set up your apartment. What room are you in?

PROTAGONIST: It's a small apartment, an efficiency. (*Shows the living-dining room, bedroom and kitchen.*)

DIRECTOR: Are you single or have you re-married?

PROTAGONIST: I am single. I have a boyfriend and we have discussed marriage but haven't made a decision.

DIRECTOR: Are you working?

PROTAGONIST: Oh, yes. I took some secretarial courses and I have a job with an insurance company.

DIRECTOR: How does it feel to be single, supporting yourself, living alone? I remember five years ago, you were very afraid of being lonely if you left Jim.

PROTAGONIST: It feels good. I'm surprised at how good it does feel. You know, what I realize now is how lonely I felt in my marriage. I am alone but not so lonely. I was at first but after I made a few friends, it was alright. I'm alright. I was silly to be so scared of loneliness. There are other things to consider but that isn't so important as I thought.

This protagonist did not want to do the alternative future projection in which she would have looked at her life five years in the future if she stayed in her marriage. However that is a possibility and may help a protagonist make a critical decision. For example, a protagonist uncertain about changing jobs or going back to school could be offered an exploration of two futures, one in which he or she dramatized both alternatives. During a future projection, the director may get cues for reenacting past scenes in the protagonist's life that will uncover residuals from old or childhood experiences that are influencing the current decision.

Death of a Significant Other

One of the common life events that often results in disequilibrium in a person's life is the death of a parent, a child, a spouse, or a relative, friend, mentor, or anybody with whom one has had an important relationship. Particularly troubling are unexpected deaths, death of a child, and, for a child, the death of a parent. The residual effects such as grief, sorrow, guilt, regret, and concerns are often dealt with in psychodrama. Moreno liked to proclaim that there is no death in psychodrama, meaning that even when they have died, people who are so important to us still influence our lives and our feelings. He also meant that we can explore our emotions and relationships, encounter these individuals who can be represented by auxiliary egos.

The following should be regarded as a very flexible outline of psychodramatizing death. Every instance is unique and requires the close attention to protagonist needs and desires. This is how I handle the psychodramatic encounter with a person who is no longer living.

If a protagonist indicates that he or she wishes to talk with a significant other who has passed away, I usually ask, "What do you think happens when we die? People have different ideas ranging from ending up in a place called heaven to the belief that dying is like turning off a light. There is nothing more. What do you believe?" This serves to warm the protagonist up to the encounter and gives me and the rest of the group information about the protagonist that is helpful in understanding the drama. A very common response to the question is that when we die there is something, a soul for some, a spirit, or essence of the person for others, that exists somewhere, somehow. For the protagonist who says that death ends all existence, I point out that there is a kind of immortality of which we can be assured, i.e., the individual exists in the memory of the protagonist and others. It is from the protagonist's memory that we will bring the individual back for an encounter. As director I also want to know when the significant other passed away.

The protagonist selects an auxiliary to take the role of the significant other. Some directors routinely ask the protagonist where they would like the encounter to take place and then set the scene. I will often suggest that we bring the significant other to the psychodrama stage and have the upcoming conversation in the here-and-now. Only if the protagonist seems to be having trouble warming up to the encounter will I suggest that we establish a setting in which to proceed. This is a time when setting a scene can either interfere with a protagonist's warm up or facilitate it. It is the director's responsibility to ascertain which course to take.

The protagonist's reason for requesting the encounter is now addressed. The encounter follows the same procedure as does any psychodramatic encounter. The protagonist states the reason for the encounter and reverses with the significant other. Soliloquy and doubling are employed when they help the protagonist in either role. The director looks for cues to events from the past involving the protagonist and the significant other and suggests psychodramatizing one or more if doing so will illuminate the relationship or help the protagonist answer questions about the relationship.

After any past events have been reenacted and the protagonist has explored the relationship to his or her satisfaction, I ask how the significant other died and if the protagonist was present at the time. Then I suggest that we reenact the death. A common situation is that the significant other died either in a hospital or in bed at home as a result of illness, an accident, or old age. This is most likely the case if the significant other is a parent or grandparent or a beloved relative, older friend, or mentor. Other possibilities include heart attacks while engaged in some activity and fatal accidents.

When the significant other has died in bed, usually from a terminal illness, the protagonist sets the scene either from memory if present at the time, or from imagination if he or she is not familiar with the actual scene. In role reversal, the director interviews the significant other. Important information is whether the significant other recognizes that he or she is dying, the status of the relationship with the protagonist, and whether the protagonist is present when the significant other dies. The director also finds out how the significant other is feeling and how he or she feels about dying.

If the protagonist was not present, the director reverses the protagonist back into his or her own role and asks if he or she would have liked to been present. If the answer is yes, which it usually is, the director indicates that we will reenact the scene as the protagonist wishes it had happened, allowing the protagonist to be with the significant other as that individual leaves life. Rarely the protagonist does not want to be present and the director allows this.

The protagonist is reversed into the role of the significant other and the director talks him or her through the act of dying. Here is an example:

The protagonist is a professional woman and is exploring the problematic relationship with her mother who died when the protagonist was 19 years old. In the drama she has produced the hypothesis that the mother resented the close relationship she and her father enjoyed. She believed that the mother felt that the father loved the daughter more than he loved the mother. The protagonist felt that she and the mother had become closer in the years before she died of cancer. The protagonist was the mother's major caretaker during her terminal illness. The scene of the mother's death has been set. The protagonist is in the bed in the role of the mother, whose name was Shirley. The protagonist and mother have exchanged feelings, both of them wishing that they had been closer earlier in the protagonist's life. The director directs the protagonist through the death of the mother.

DIRECTOR: Alright, Shirley, the time has come for you to leave this life. I know that it has not been a particularly easy life and that you are dying rather young.

MOTHER (P): Yes.

DIRECTOR: Be aware of your body and how it feels. *(Pause.)* Soon you will feel your life energy ebbing away. Just be aware of it. As it decreases, at some point, you will be aware that you have crossed the line between being alive and being dead. Let me know when you know that you have crossed that line by moving a finger. *(Waits until protagonist indicates as directed.)* How does it feel to be dead?

MOTHER (P): *(Slow to answer and in a very soft, voice)* Peaceful. Calm.

DIRECTOR: Calm and peaceful?

MOTHER (P): Yes.

DIRECTOR: No more pain, is there?

MOTHER (P): No.

DIRECTOR: Do you feel light or heavy?

MOTHER (P): Light.

DIRECTOR: Does it seem light or dark?

MOTHER (P): Dark.

DIRECTOR: Do you have a sense of movement?

MOTHER (P): Not really.

DIRECTOR: Do you have a sense of anybody or any entity with you?

MOTHER (P): No.

DIRECTOR: (*Allows the protagonist some time to experience the state that she is in.)*

Then I would like you to reverse roles. Take your time. Open your eyes. Don't rush to sit up.

PROTAGONIST: *(Slowly sits up and reverses roles with the auxiliary mother.)*

DIRECTOR: Hold her hand if you wish as she leaves us, or put your head on her shoulder. Is there anything more you wish to say?

PROTAGONIST: *(Holds mother's hand. Softly)* Goodbye. I do love you. *(Weeps briefly.)*

DIRECTOR: *(Waits until protagonist looks up.)* Shall we let her go to wherever it is in the cosmos that she now belongs?

PROTAGONIST: Yes.

It can't be emphasized too strongly that guiding a protagonist through this procedure requires spontaneity and the utmost sensitivity to the protagonist on the part of the director. Death is a powerfully emotional issue and the director must be ready to respond to any need of the protagonist who is experiencing the death of a significant other. I believe that one should experience the psychodramatization of dying as a protagonist before attempting to direct it. Zerka Moreno suggested that psychodrama directors should all have the experience of dramatizing their own deaths. Other approaches to dealing with death in psychodrama can be found in Siroka & Schloss, (1968; Abraham, 1972).

In 1973, Ernest Becker (1973), cultural anthropologist, published the book, *Denial of Death*, the theme of which was that fear of death is universal among human beings, and is a major motivator of human activity, the aim of which is to deny that death is the final destiny for man. Fear of death is certainly widespread if not universal. Protagonists report that the psychodramatic experience of death is a profound one and leaves them feeling more accepting, less fearful of death. *For that reason, one should never consider psychodramatizing death with a protagonist who has expressed any hint of suicidal thinking.* Doing so could serve to warm the individual up to committing the act. The exception to this caveat is discussed in the section on dealing with suicide.

The questions that I ask about the experience of death are based on statements that protagonists have spontaneously made in describing their psychodramatic experiences of death. I routinely ask the questions to assist protagonists in exploring the experience. Some protagonists report feeling light, others feel heavy. It is the same with the other questions. Some people report darkness, others lightness, and some see a white light. Occasionally a protagonist will report sensing the presence of a parent, a child, or someone else who has preceded them in death. A few have felt the presence of God or Jesus.

I have met people who have trained with other psychodrama trainers who tell me that they have been taught to never psychodramatize death. That is certainly a safe position to take but J. L. Moreno proclaimed that the practice of psychodrama required courage. That position is also counter to what I learned and taught at the Moreno Institute, although it is worth repeating that one should have the experience before directing it, and that it should never be attempted when suicide is concerned.

Decision Making

Future projection has been presented as a way of helping an individual explore alternative courses of action when faced with a major life decision. When a protagonist is still feeling uncertain about which choice to make after a lengthy exploration, or if a person is vacillating between two choices over an issue that does not seem to warrant a long exploration, the following procedures may be helpful.

The protagonist is directed to divide the stage. One side will represent one course of action; the other side represents the alternative. The protagonist picks an auxiliary to represent the first choice. A role reversal is called and the protagonist in the role of the first choice gives all the reasons he or she can think of for the protagonist to select it. An auxiliary is chosen to represent the other choice. In role reversal, the protagonist gives all the reasons why this choice should be picked. The protagonist in her or his role then stands between the two and listens to the auxiliaries, each urging the protagonist to choose that option.

This externalization of the protagonist's inner thoughts may resolve the dilemma for the protagonist. If it doesn't, the next step is a concretization of being pulled in two directions. The protagonist stands between the two auxiliaries, extending her or his arms. Each auxiliary takes one arm and, at the word of the director, pulls the protagonist toward their side of the stage. At the same time, the auxiliaries repeat the advantages that the protagonist has earlier produced. The director gives instructions on how hard to pull, gently at first, then harder. Eventually, the protagonist is very likely to begin pulling in one direction or the other. Often, the director and the group members will see the protagonist lean in one direction or the other early in the exercise, before the protagonist is aware of having that preference.

Suicide Psychodrama

It was in 1921, according to biographer Marineau (1989) and J. D. Moreno (2014), while he was the village doctor in Voslau and before he had used spontaneity theater techniques for treatment of marital problems, that Moreno dealt with a suicidal man. The patient was wealthy but not happy and his request was for Moreno to help him commit suicide. Moreno agreed to help him. He then started a course of treatment, entering the man's inner world. For weeks they talked about planning death: the man wrote his last will, discussed at length different ways of killing himself, ate with renewed appetite knowing that it might be his last meal, and acted out different scenarios. He did this with the assistance of Moreno and Moreno's partner, Marianne.

I heard a version of the story from Martin Haskell early in my training. According to Haskell, the climax came when Moreno decided that it was time to rehearse the suicide itself. A method was chosen. The patient acted it out, eventually dying psychodramatically. Now, Moreno told the "dead" man, the problem is the body. There should be a funeral. The patient agreed and so the scene was set—by the patient. Moreno had him role reverse with each of the attendees, then with the patient in his coffin asked, "Is there anyone with whom you would like to speak?"

"Yes," the man replied, "I would like to talk with my father."

"Of course you can't do that now that you are dead," Moreno told him, and paused. "But if you were to choose life instead of death, you could speak to your father." According to Haskell, the patient chose to live.

Psychodramatically enacting suicide carries a major risk, Moreno warned. "The psychodramatic realization of suicidal or homicidal fantasies may give courage and prepare a patient to carry out the suicide in life itself," Moreno wrote (1973, p. 23). If it is not carried out correctly, psychodrama can could actually serve as role training and warm the client up to completing the act. The aim of a suicide psychodrama is prophylaxis, to prevent the client from taking their own life. This is accomplished by confronting the protagonist with the impact of their death on the significant others whom they leave behind. The following drama, illustrating this principle, took place in a personal growth psychodrama workshop:

The protagonist is a woman in her early 30s. Her husband has divorced her less than a year ago and she has an eight year old son. She has been struggling psychologically and economically, and feels fatigued and like a total failure. She blames herself for the husband leaving; she was not an adequate wife and mother. The only way she sees for obtaining some peace is to end her life.

DIRECTOR: Have you considered how you would end your life?

PROTAGONIST: Oh, yes. I have sat and looked at the bottle of aspirin for an hour at a time.

DIRECTOR: I see. Well, let's see what would happen. When and where do you imagine yourself swallowing enough aspirin to kill yourself?

PROTAGONIST: In the kitchen.

DIRECTOR: Take us there. *(Protagonist sets the scene.)* What time is it?

PROTAGONIST: It's night-time, say 11 o'clock.

DIRECTOR: Show us what you do. *(Protagonist goes through the motions of taking bottle out of cabinet and taking several handfuls of pills, drinking water with each bunch. She sits down at the table and lays her head down on one arm.)* And how long is it before you begin to feel the effects?

PROTAGONIST: I think I get drowsy after about 20 or 30 minutes.

DIRECTOR: *(After a long pause of perhaps a minute or two.)* O. K. Let's go to the point where you get drowsy. *(Long pause.)* And after some more time, you begin to feel your life energy leaving your body. Let yourself feel that. Let me know when you have crossed over the border between life and death. Let me know by raising a finger on your right hand. *(Waits. After a while, protagonist signals.)* Now you are dead. How does it feel to be dead. You can answer even if you are dead.

PROTAGONIST: It is very peaceful. I feel calm and relaxed. Very relaxed.

DIRECTOR: *(Allows the protagonist to remain quiet until some movement suggests that it is time to go on.)* And who finds your body?

PROTAGONIST: *(Sits up.)* Timmy, I guess.

DIRECTOR: Alright, it's morning. Reverse roles with your son, Timmy.

PROTAGONIST: (*Begins to cry.*) No. (*Sobs.*) I don't want to. I can't!

DIRECTOR: I know. I understand that you don't want to. But I think it will be helpful for if you will do this.

PROTAGONIST: O. K. I'll try. *(Timmy's bedroom is located on part of the stage. A double selected earlier in the drama takes the role of the protagonist sitting at the kitchen table with her head on her arm.)*

DIRECTOR: Timmy. It's morning and you wake up show us what you do.

"TIMMY" (P): I get out of bed and go down to the kitchen to have breakfast. (*Goes into kitchen. Sees mother and goes to her.*) Mother, are you asleep? (*Shakes her. Then begins to cry. Director helps her to the floor where she curls up and wails and sobs for minutes. It becomes evident that she has dropped out of the role of Timmy and is crying for herself. Director encourages her expression of pain which goes on and on. Her hurt is so evident and palpable that most of the group members are weeping or tearful as well. The director is patient and waits until the sobbing has subsided.*)

PROTAGONIST: *(In a quiet voice.)* I could never do that to him.

The director believes that the psychodrama has served its purpose. The protagonist is completely worn out and the group is feeling emotionally depleted as well. The director invites the group members to join him and the protagonist, who are sitting on the floor of the stage, for sharing.

The Magic Shop

The magic shop is a fantasy exercise in which a number of group members can have a brief protagonist experience. The shop itself has a wide and unusual inventory of items, all of which are intangible. One can shop here for insight, peace of mind, joy, wisdom, patience, assertiveness, almost any trait, quality, or personality characteristic one can imagine. Of course these items cannot be purchased with money. Rather, one barters with the shopkeeper, giving up one quality or trait in return for the desired one The shopkeeper decides if what the customer wishes to give up is valuable enough to exchange for what the customer desires.

The exercise goes like this: A shopkeeper is designated and can be the director or any member of the group. The role can be passed around during the exercise. The shopkeeper describes the shop, him or herself, and perhaps the location of the shop. The shopkeeper can be an old, wizened elf or crone, a fairy-like creature, or anything the shopkeeper cares to imagine. The shop may be "just around the corner" or under a large oak tree, according to the desires of the shopkeeper who also describes the shop, large or small with shelves or drawers, or perhaps the inventory is kept in the back room. Some shopkeepers have an assistant who helps them with the bargaining in various ways.

Once the shopkeeper has set the scene group members are invited to enter, shop and barter for their heart's desire. Group members enter the shop one by one, state what they want and decide in interaction with the shopkeeper what they will give up. Example:

Customer enters the magic shop.

SHOPKEEPER: How can I help you.

CUSTOMER: I'm not sure. I would just like to look around. Just what is you have here?

SHOPKEEPER: We have 'most anything a person could want. Is there anyway you think you would like to be different than you are?

CUSTOMER: Well, yes. During this workshop, I found myself wishing that I could be more open with people. Like some of the other people in the workshop.

SHOPKEEPER: Openness. I see. Yes, we could provide some Openness for you. What would you give me in return?

CUSTOMER: Gosh, I am not sure. *(Pauses to think.)* I could give you some of my anxiety.

SHOPKEEPER: Anxiety? Well, I've got a pretty big container of anxiety in the back. Don't get much call for that. How about something else?

CUSTOMER: I am pretty intelligent. I guess I could give you some of my intelligence.

SHOPKEEPER: I certainly could sell that easily. But to tell you the truth, I'm not sure that you should give any of your intelligence away, event for Openness. *(Both are quiet, thinking. Then)*

How about security? There's a demand for that. Would you give me some security in return for some Openness with others?

CUSTOMER: *(Seems taken aback by Shopkeeper's suggestion.)* I'm not sure I want to give up my security.

SHOPKEEPER: It's valuable. You don't need to give me much. How about a little Openness in return for a little security?

CUSTOMER: (*After a pause to think it over.*) Well, O. K. I guess I will.

Hanna Weiner, a star of the psychodrama collective from the 1950s through the 1970s, was considered a master of the magic shop. She demonstrated her spontaneity as the shopkeeper as well as the dynamics of the magic shop in a session in which I participated in 1962.

The customer is a young, energetic woman beginning her training in psychodrama.

CUSTOMER: I would like to have more patience.
SHOPKEEPER: Sit down there while I take care of this next customer.
CUSTOMER: But … *(Starts to say, "But I was here first," then realizes that the shopkeeper has given her an opportunity to practice what she has asked for.)*

The magic shop most often occurs during the course of multi-session workshop although it has been used in client groups to good advantage. It is effective both for an opening session and a closing session, serving as either a warming up to a workshop or a closure exercise. Some directors employ the magic shop when a group is low energy or as a relief after the group has engaged in several intensive psychodrama sessions. Many books on psychodrama describe the magic shop and Barbour (1992) has written a thoughtful article on the subject.

Role Training

Role training is a method of teaching or enhancing social skills. Role training is likely the most widely applied psychodrama format although a majority of those who use it are unaware of its psychodramatic origins. A role training sequence may be introduced into therapeutic or personal growth psychodrama to help a protagonist better take a real life role. It has been used to teach groups how to handle a common problem. Servicemen with psychiatric problems who were admitted to St. Elizabeth Hospital after World War II underwent a role training procedure prior to their discharge. These former servicemen were often hospitalized for many months and in this time, psychiatric hospitalization was decidedly stigmatized. The role training was established to help them figure out how to answer the questions of neighbors, relatives, prospective employers, etc. about the period in which they were patients at St. Elizabeth Hospital.

Role training has been utilized to teach the complex set of social skills that serve to establish the professional identity of nurses, physicians, and lawyers. Under the title of role playing, role training has been widely applied in business and industry to teach supervisory and administrative skills. Role training has to do with human relations, ethical values, and attitudes.

J. L. Moreno introduced role training into New York State Training School for Girls at Hudson to deal with the responsibility of that institution to prepare delinquent teenage girls to live independently in open society after their discharge from the school at age 18. Moreno undertook to fulfill this task by training them for the kinds of jobs they were likely to find when they left the school, clerks in stores, waitresses in restaurants, and the like. He conducted training sessions in which the group members took the roles of waitress, for example, and customers. The customers ordered, the waitresses served. The customers posed various problem situations such as complaining about food, waiting too long, etc., for the waitresses to deal with. The group then critiqued the waitress's performance and made suggestions on how she could improve. Sociologist Martin Haskell, one of the early master psychodramatists, was a strong proponent of role training and played a major role in introducing role training in business and industry. Haskell (M. R. Haskell, 1957, 1959), and others (R. J. Haskell & Larr, 1974), have written a number of articles on the subject.

A number of psychodramatic techniques are used in role training. Usually the protagonist is allowed to play the role as he or she has done in the past or anticipates or imagines doing in the future. In a role reversal with the complementary person or persons, the protagonist's performance, both verbal and body language, is mirrored by an auxiliary. In this way the protagonist critiques his or her own behavior. The protagonist is allowed to play the role in as many ways as desired. Soliloquy in both roles produces the underlying emotional response to the performance. The director, after the protagonist has rehearsed the situation thoroughly, may choose to ask the other members of the group to demonstrate how they would handle the situation that the protagonist has presented. The protagonist takes the role of the significant other. This maneuver is especially helpful when the protagonist is preparing for a problematic situation such as confronting a supervisor with the supervisor's unethical behavior. After group members have acted out their solutions to the situation, the protagonist is invited to reenact the situation again, this time incorporating any ideas that the group has provided.

A relatively complete role training procedure for preparing a person to apply for a job might include the following steps:

1. A trained auxiliary takes the role of a prospective employer. The situation will be one that is realistic with respect to the protagonist and the type of position for which the protagonist might reasonably apply.
2. The scene of the interview is set. Perhaps there is a receptionist (taken by an auxiliary) to whom the job applicant announces him or herself. The employer asks the receptionist to send in the applicant.
3. The employer interviews the applicant.
4. The applicant then reverses roles with the employer. The interview is reenacted. The auxiliary responds as closely as possible to the way the applicant initially answers the employer's questions.
5. Still in the role of the employer, the applicant evaluates the applicant as played by the auxiliary. If there are criticisms of the applicant, the director calls for a role reversal and invites the trainee, now in the applicant role, to redo those parts of the interview that he or she was not satisfied with when in the employer role.

6. This procedure is repeated until the applicant is satisfied with his or her own performance.
7. If role training is being carried out in a group, after the individual has exhausted his or her responses to the situation, the director may invite group members to demonstrate how they would manage the situation. In this case, the protagonist is put into the role of the employer so that he or she can evaluate these responses from that position.

After all group members have been given an opportunity to act, the trainee is invited to pick and choose any (or none) of the elements of their responses and incorporate them into his or her performance.

The director uses soliloquy whenever it may be helpful for the protagonist to think out loud. For example, the receptionist asks the applicant to sit down and wait until the prospective employer calls for him or her. The director may ask for a soliloquy to determine whether the protagonist is anxious, confident, anticipatory or whatever he or she is feeling. A soliloquy might be called for if the applicant is hesitating as well as when the protagonist is in the role of the employer. Doubling may also be called for to help the protagonist identify and articulate feelings in either role.

Action Social Atom

The social atom is a concept from sociometry, Moreno's theory of society. A social atom consists of an individual and all other people with whom that individual has a meaningful relationship. Also included in one's social atom are individuals with whom one wants a meaningful relationship as well as others who would like a relationship with the individual. A social atom, rather than an individual, is the smallest unit of society. We are more often interested in an individual's social atom with respect to one of the collectives to which that person belongs. Thus, we speak of one's family social atom, or one's workplace social atom, or of one's social atom with respect to an organization such as a church or social club. A social atom is typically represented by a sociogram, a graphic device depicting the individual and each member of the social atom. An action sociogram is a psychodramatic device in which the protagonist uses auxiliaries to represent the significant others in his or her life. Barbara Seabourne (1963) has written an article on the action sociogram.

The action social atom is used to explore in depth the protagonist's social atom. It adds action techniques such as role reversal and soliloquy to a paper and pencil social atom exploration. The action social atom begins with asking the protagonist to locate on the stage the protagonist's place in the social group under consideration, the family, for instance. Once the protagonist's place has been designated and taken by the protagonist, the protagonist is asked to identify the person towards whom the protagonist has the strongest feelings, positive or negative, and to place that person where he or she belongs relative to the protagonist. An auxiliary ego is chosen by the protagonist to portray that individual and the protagonist makes a statement to the significant other about their relationship. A role reversal ensues and as the significant other, the protagonist responds to the statement. If the significant other's feelings toward the protagonist are not clear, the director asks the protagonist-in-role-of-significant other to state those feelings.

The protagonist reversed back into self and identifies the next most important person in the social atom, make a statement, role reverse and respond, etc. This continues until the protagonist has identified all the others in this social atom.

At this point, the protagonist is on stage with auxiliaries playing the roles of all the others in the social atom. The director has a number of choices. One is to have each auxiliary repeat the statement that was originally assigned to the role. The protagonist can be asked if he or she would like to make any changes in his or her social atom. The protagonist may reply that he or she would like to be closer to one or more of the significant others, or would like to increase the distance of others. The director can then ask the protagonist what would be required to bring those changes about and allow the protagonist to explore those actions psychodramatically. Frequently, an action social atom leads to encounters with one or more of the significant others and possibly further psychodramatic action. The possibilities are limited only by the director's and the protagonist's creativity.

Family Psychodrama

Given Moreno's interpersonal perception of psychological problems, it makes sense that he was a pioneer in family therapy as well as in the treatment of marital difficulties (Compernolle, 1981). Moreno made use of both sociometric ideas as well as the action methods in assisting families to resolve their problems and develop effective ways of interacting. An illustrative chapter by Zerka Moreno (1991) gives a detailed account of her work with a blended family of eight persons. The family consists of mother and father in a second marriage, and their children from their respective first marriages, five from the father's and one from the mother's. The entire family came to the Moreno Institute where they stayed and had nine sessions in the psychodrama theater. Zerka gives an account of each session, describing the interactions of various the family members, the conclusions drawn from them, and the decisions for change made. The psychodramatic literature has many citations for family psychodrama, sociodrama, and the use of psychodramatic techniques in family therapy based on different methods.

Improvisation

Because psychodrama evolved from Moreno's spontaneity theater, it is not surprising that he introduced several improvisational procedures into the method. These include spontaneity testing, the role playing test, the situation test, and spontaneity training (J. L. Moreno, 1953b). The role training process described above also fits into this category. All of these procedures involve assigning a role to the individual being tested or trained and asking them to play out a situation, usually with an auxiliary ego. The situations involve conflict; for example, the subject is assigned the role of an employee who is being fired for coming in to work late, or a boyfriend who is accused of being unfaithful by his girlfriend. Sometimes an auxiliary is not required. For instance, the subject is in his home when he smells smoke and discovers a fire has broken out in one part of the house. He is informed that there is an infant in one bedroom and important papers in another part of the house, and someone is approaching the house to enter near the location of the fire. As Moreno pointed out, whether it is a role test or a spontaneity test depends upon what the administrator of the test is investigating. When the situation was to explore the subject's ability to mobilize sufficient spontaneity in playing out imaginary or lifelike situations, it was a spontaneity test. When the purpose was to assess the range of roles and adequacy in playing them, it was role testing. Situation testing could guide further training for life skills. All served as spontaneity training.

Moreno used these instruments extensively in his reconstruction of the Hudson Training School society. He also illustrated their use in marital therapy in *Psychodrama, First Volume* (1946b). He reports working with a couple, Robert and Mary. Robert has a serious anxiety disorder and it is complicated by marital problems. Moreno assigns them a series of role relationships, such as sheriff and shoplifter and district attorney interrogating a suspect criminal, that they are instructed to enact on the stage. The purpose is partially diagnostic and partially to increase their spontaneity in relation to each other. Improvisation allows an individual to experience psychodramatic roles, roles that they would like to play in life but cannot for various reasons including social pressures or lack of opportunity. Today, improvisation is utilized less frequently by psychodramatists. Improvisational theater training, however, makes extensive use of such exercises.

Post-Traumatic Stress

Life circumstances confront some people with monumentally disturbing events, experiences in which there is a threat to one's life or physical integrity. Exposure to war as a combatant or civilian, threatened or actual physical assault, physical attack, robbery, mugging, childhood physical abuse, threatened or actual sexual violence being kidnapped or taken hostage, terrorist attack, torture, incarceration as a prisoner of war, natural or human-made disasters, and severe motor vehicle accidents are examples. Experiences such as these can have serious, long term deleterious effects on one's well-being, a situation which is called post-traumatic stress disorder, abbreviated PTSD. Death, harm, or threat of harm to others, one's children or other close relations especially, can also precipitate the condition. Sexual abuse of children, even when there is no physical violence or injury, is a common origin of PTSD that often results in dissociation and persists into adulthood. Sigmund Freud's original theory of the etiology of hysteria was that it resulted from the trauma of childhood sexual seduction, frequently by the father. He later disavowed this hypothesis. Childhood seduction and rape, however, are today considered major sources of post-traumatic stress disorder.

The residual effects of such experiences include unwanted recall of the traumatic event along with the emotions and thoughts that accompanied it and dreams in which the event is replicated. Some individuals experience flashbacks in which they feel as if the event is actually happening again. Difficulty in sleeping and in concentration, irritability, constricted affect, and dissociative phenomena can occur as well.

The designation as post-traumatic stress disorder was established in the 1970's in response to the emotional problems of veterans of the Vietnam wars although the phenomenon has been recognized at least throughout the twentieth century. The American Psychiatric Association's description is found in its *Diagnostic and statistical manual of mental disorders* (2015). It is considered to be the latest formulation of the condition called shell shock in World War I and battle fatigue in World War II. Because of the great numbers of veterans of the Vietnam and Middle East wars, PTSD has received extensive attention from the mental health professions. It has proven to be a condition that is difficult to ameliorate. Current thought holds that exposure to overwhelming trauma causes neurological changes in the brain. Irish psychiatrist, Ivor Browne, proposes a more psycho-biological explanation for PTSD. I will discuss that in the chapter on theory.

Psychodrama provides one of the most effective ways of helping people cope with the events that result in PTSD. It requires, however, a careful and delicate touch by the director. This is an area where improper procedures can result in re-traumatization of the protagonist instead of healing. Nowhere is Moreno's dictum that a psychodrama should start at the periphery of the issue being explored and move toward the center more important. In working with an individual with PTSD, the director does not begin by dramatizing the traumatic event. As a matter of fact, a number of sessions may occur before such a scene is attempted. Thus, a veteran whose trauma includes the loss of good friends, a common situation, may begin by psychodramatic encounters with one or more of them, expressing grief, guilt at not being able to protect them or for having survived when they did not, or any of a multitude of emotions associated with them. These scenes are deeply touching and afford considerable relief to the protagonists. Another possibility is the expression of anger to incompetent leadership or to someone perceived as responsible for putting the protagonist in the situation. With the protagonist who has been sexually, physically, or emotionally abused as a child, the first scene may be a confrontation of the abuser. If it is difficult for the protagonist to do this with an auxiliary ego in the role of the abuser, an empty chair in which the protagonist pictures the abuser may be used.

Dramatization of the traumatic event or events can be gradually approached. Rather than reenacting the event themselves, protagonists may be allowed to describe what happened while auxiliaries act it out. The protagonist watches from off stage as auxiliaries enact the scene from the protagonist's description of it. This is the incorporation of Jonathan Fox's Playback Theater process. During such a reenactment, the director may observe the protagonist warming up to his or her own role or to the role of someone else in the drama, perhaps an abuser, and can invite the protagonist to enter the enactment. Eventually the protagonist will be able to reenact the occurrence him or herself. It is important that the protagonist reverse roles with the abuser, if there the trauma involves abuse. This may take some time for the traumatized protagonist to accomplish. A common question that the protagonist will have is "Why did this happen to me?" It can require a lot of ingenuity and creativity on the part of the director to help the protagonist resolve this question.

Individuals who have been abused as children often cope during abuse by dissociating. As protagonists in psychodramas, they sometimes soliloquize something like, "This is not me that this is happening to" when the abuse is being reenacted. In a psychodrama of abuse, dissociation as the protagonist warms up to the actual scene of abuse can be a problem for the director. During dissociation, the protagonist becomes minimally responsive even to the point of seeming catatonic. The drama cannot continue when the protagonist becomes unresponsive to the director, the auxiliaries, and the psychodramatic situation. It is also quite alarming to group members unfamiliar with the state so directors like to avoid it. The experienced director can usually detect that the protagonist is warming up to dissociation and intervene by taking the protagonist out of the scene. Hudgens (2002) has developed a structured approach to the psychodramatizing of trauma, which is designed to reduce the likelihood of dissociation.

Psychodrama of Meaningful Experiences

Moreno contended that every important event in a person's life should be experienced at least twice, once when it occurred, and at least once on the psychodrama stage. The vast majority of psychodramas involve experiences of the protagonist that involve negative emotions, largely interpersonal interactions that have not gone as the protagonist anticipated or wished. These events have left the protagonist frustrated, hurt, angry, or at least puzzled and wondering why things turned out as they did. A successful psychodrama allows the protagonist to express the emotions that recall of the experience re-activates, as well as to understand more fully why the interaction played out as it did instead of the way that the protagonist expected. People also have powerful positive experiences also, and psychodramatization of these events has a beneficial impact upon both the protagonist and the group.

I have written an account of such psychodramas under the title, *Protagonist without a Problem*, (Nolte, 2008) and have presented the psychodrama of a meaningful experience at several conferences. Themes of positive psychodramas include giving birth, falling in love, receiving special or unexpected gifts, both material and immaterial, triumphs, and relationships between grandparents and grandchildren. I have used the psychodramatization of positive experiences to demonstrate the psychodrama method to groups in which it seemed inappropriate to ask someone to engage in a typical, problem oriented psychodramatic exploration. The method and all its techniques can be demonstrated in this way without danger of embarrassing or exposing the protagonist.

Psychodramatic Rite of Passage

A special case of psychodrama that is not problem centered is a psychodrama that is produced in order to celebrate a change in status. Students of psychodrama who have achieved certification sometimes are protagonists in psychodramas, the aim of which is to memorialize the achievement. These often involve the identification of significant and noteworthy events in their journey toward becoming psychodrama directors. These become the events in the psychodrama of celebration.

Another example of this type of psychodrama occurred when a mother of a young woman who was soon departing for college asked for a psychodrama to help both of them cope with the separation as well as to celebrate the daughter's new status. The mother had been single when the daughter was born and the two had become quite close as they struggled with life's problems for the ensuing 18 years. They invited friends to make up the group. The psychodrama began with the mother, 19 years old, bringing home from the hospital the brand new baby. Single and estranged from her parents, she soliloquized her fears, her feelings of inadequacies about being a mother, as well as her commitment to the new life she had brought into the world. From there, mother and daughter reenacted experiences that marked their journey together, each taking turns at identifying scenes to be re-experienced. The drama concluded with an encounter in which each expressed their concerns, hopes, and wishes, for themselves and for each other.

Adjunct Methods

In her important article on guidelines, rules, and techniques, Zerka Moreno (1965) lists several adjunctive methods that are seldom used today. These include psychodramatic shock treatment, hypnodrama, didactic psychodrama, and psychodrama combined with narcosynthesis, LSD, etc. I include a brief description of these methods for completion and as a historical note.

Psychodramatic Shock Treatment

J. L. Moreno (1939) published an article on this subject in an early issue of *Sociometry*. The technique is used with psychotic patients. Shortly after a psychotic episode, when the individual is lucid, he or she is encouraged "to throw himself back into the psychotic world. This upsetting experience is called 'psychodramatic shock'" (p. 1). With the help of auxiliaries to represent hallucinations and other creations of the psychotic experience, the individual does so but with the control of the experience that psychodrama provides. According to Moreno, psychodramatic shock treatment serves as a research method for better understanding of mental disorders, and simultaneously has a cathartic effect upon the patient.

Hypnodrama

J. L. Moreno introduced this combination of hypnosis and psychodrama in an article published in 1950. Moreno was working with a delusional patient who dreamed that every night the devil came to visit her. She was unable to psychodramatize these events. However, in one session she spontaneously went into a hypnotic trance. In this state, she was able to reenact, with the aid of auxiliaries, two meetings that she had with the devil. Moreno reports that he then tried hypnotizing other subjects who could not otherwise muster sufficient spontaneity to engage in psychodramatic activity. He reported that the method was often successful. Enneis (1943) discusses the use of hypnodrama in another article, outlining the steps in its application. He presents a hypnodramatic session with a young man diagnosed as paranoid schizophrenia whose psychodramatic work had been characterized by sluggish movement and difficulty in speaking.

Hypnodrama does not seem to be a very widely used method. Although there are about a dozen articles in the literature, four of them are in Greenberg's (1977) book on hypnotherapy and hypnodrama. With the exception of two other articles in German, the others were all published by 1967. One of the reasons why hypnosis with protagonists is relatively rare is that, as Moreno pointed out, few people actually resist psychodrama. Although at a time early in my career as a psychotherapist, I studied and trained in hypnotherapy,

I gave it up as soon as I began working with psychodrama, preferring the more equal, collaborative relationship between director and protagonist to the seemingly unequal relationship of hypnotherapist and patient.

Didactic Psychodrama

A wide variety of activities can be subsumed under this heading ranging from teaching psychodrama skills to the use of action methods in teaching conventional subjects. Role training and bibliodrama can be placed under this classification. I was invited to conduct in-service training sessions for the nurses of a general hospital, where I was on the psychiatric staff, from time to time. I usually started the session by asking the group to identify the biggest problem the nursing staff faced. We then used reenactment to illustrate the problem and to seek possible solutions. Depending upon the problem that was presented, the nurses played the roles of patients, supervisors, administration, doctors or visitors. After enacting situations that illustrated the problem, psychodramatic brainstorming followed. Every possibility for resolution that the group could come up with was tried out.

I once conducted a workshop with the staff of a school of nursing with the aim of looking for ways of using action methods in their teaching duties. The most obvious applications involved social skills ranging from nurse-patient relationships to teacher-student relationships. However, in one session, the group developed a way of teaching the electrical circuitry of the heart, in action. It was the conclusion of the group that participating in that exercise would likely be far more effective in understanding and remembering the subject matter than would lecture and drawings on the chalk board.

Psychodrama techniques have been used in literature and history classes as well. Acting out the stories, whether they are the fiction of literature or interpretations of historical events adds a dimension that goes far beyond that possible with only words. Reenactment also gives participants in the process an experience beyond that of even the most artistic theatrical presentation. Putting oneself in the role of historical and fictional characters provides an experience far more meaningful than watching the most talented actor portray it.

Psychodrama Combined with Narcosynthesis, LSD, and Insulin

Although Moreno was generally very cautious about the use of drugs, he does mention the use of alcohol, sodium pentothal, and insulin as potential starters or warm ups (J. L. Moreno, 1953b). He also published an article on combining sub-shock doses of insulin with psychodrama in the treatment of psychotic patients with positive results (J. L. Moreno & Schwartz, 1948). Although Rackow (1951) reported on using this combination of insulin and psychodrama and a number of other activities with 98 patients at a Veterans Administration Hospital in New York, I find no evidence that this ever became a widely used approach.

Moreno was also persuaded by a colleague who was experimenting with LSD and psychotherapy to bring a group to the Moreno Institute. There the effects of the drug on psychodrama were studied. The results were chaos and the experiment was never repeated (J. D. Moreno, 2014).

Strategies of Directing

The concept of strategies of directing developed from my observations of experienced directors during the years when I was first learning the method. Watching the stars of the psychodramatic collective of those days, directors including Zerka Moreno, Jim Enneis, Martin Haskell, Hannah Weiner, Lew Yablonsky, Adaline Starr and Leon Fine and others, I was puzzled by the big differences in the how each went about directing a psychodrama. Yet each drama was none the less effective. I was frustrated because I was trying to learn the *correct* way to direct.

I discussed my puzzlement with Moreno. He suggested that the differences I saw were related to his differing styles of directing at the time the individual was a student. Although J. L. Moreno taught that directors of psychodrama develop individual styles, it seemed to me that more was involved. I noticed both similarities and differences.

As I pondered on these matters, it gradually occurred to me that what I was attending to were different patterns, different ways in which directors formulated and approached the problems presented by their protagonists. Here is where the life experiences of the director interacted with the life experiences of the protagonist. Although the notion of a strategy may seem to be inconsistent in the context of spontaneity methods, this is not really so. Though neither the protagonist nor the director knows at the beginning of drama just what will emerge or how the drama will turn out, there are elements of planning and organization which the director utilizes in the task of co-producing the psychodrama. These include some of the factors I call strategies of directing. A strategy will be influenced by the director's understanding and perception of psychodrama as a method and how the director perceives its use as a therapeutic instrument. Also involved is the director's philosophy and understanding of human nature, as well as the director's understanding of psychopathology and emotional disequilibrium. Most directors utilize several strategies in their work, moving from one to another in response to the protagonist and the themes which the protagonist presents. I have identified several strategies which appear to be fairly common within the psychodrama collective. There may be other major strategies and an infinite number of variations on each one. A strategy is not identical to personal style but is inextricably bound up with the director's style

Four strategies of directing are described below. I have observed each of these in the work of experienced psychodrama trainers and nationally recognized leaders in the fields. Many of the observations from which this concept is derived were made at the annual psychodrama conferences. I call the strategies the psychodynamic strategy; the sociometric strategy; the psychodramatic strategy; and the sociodramatic strategy.

The Psychodynamic Strategy

This is an approach toward which many of us, who were originally trained in traditional forms of psychotherapy, naturally gravitate, and which we probably utilize initially we become familiar with all the possibilities that psychodrama offers. This strategy emphasizes the therapist role of the director and the patient role of the protagonist in a traditional manner. The protagonist is perceived as having a problem or symptoms of a disorder, and the director is perceived as an expert who has techniques that will resolve the issue. The problem will likely be construed in terms of the protagonist's internal dynamics and conflicts.

The director who relies heavily upon this strategy will often direct dramas in which there is a lot of intrapersonal psychodrama. That is, he will have the protagonist confronting or encountering parts of self, his anger, his fear, his depression, etc. He may dramatize internal conflicts using the double ego technique with doubles representing various aspects of the conflict.

Of course there are many other systems of internal dynamics besides the psychoanalytic one to which the term psychodynamic usually refers. If the director using this strategy has been trained in transactional analysis, for example, he may produce the protagonist's parent, adult, and child ego states. If an encounter is involved, the director may produce the ego states of both parties. The more sophisticated psychodramatist-sociometrician will cast these issues as role conflicts, and will deal with role-rigidity or over-conserved roles. A major characteristic of this strategy is its focus on fixing something internal, something within the protagonist which is interfering in the protagonist's life.

The Sociometric Strategy

This is a social systems approach, and begins to be incorporated by many new directors as they become acquainted with the sociometric aspects of Morenean theory. The director whose style incorporates this strategy will attend carefully to the social environment of the protagonist. If, as frequently happens, the protagonist produces a scene in his home, current or past, this director will find out exactly who else is living here, assign these roles to auxiliaries, and get some degree of the family dynamics into the action. If the scene is at the office, we will learn something of the protagonist's work social atom.

This strategy shifts from emphasis from intra-personal conflict to interpersonal relationships in a social context. Social investigation is a frequent activity of this strategy, carried out through role-reversal and use of auxiliaries. The director aims at understanding the protagonist's from the perspective of the protagonist's sociometric position in a specific group setting. The main characteristic of this strategy is producing sociometric data and social dynamics in the drama. This is an approach that is quite useful in psychodramatic family therapy.

The Psychodramatic Strategy

In both the sociometric strategy and the psychodramatic strategy, psychopathology is minimized. Many directors move easily from one of these strategies to the other. The orientation of the psychodramatic strategy is telling a story in action. The story is an event in the protagonist's life, present or past, or a fantasy, a dream, or an ambition. In the process, the protagonist's thoughts and emotions are elicited during the dramatic presentation of the content. Well done, the psychodrama should make apparent to all who take part in it that the protagonist is showing to the group members that "This is what it is like to be me, to live my life."

The director using this strategy will think in terms of story more than analyzing the psychological dynamics of the protagonist. Of course, the perceptions and motivations of those with whom the protagonist interacts, referred to as significant others, are important aspects of the protagonist's story, and are elicited through role reversal and active auxiliary work. Some stories can be told in a single scene but more often this strategy produces several. The director will also be encouraging protagonists to produce not only what may have happened before, but to expand upon the original, to express the feelings which were not or could not be expressed in the real-life experience. They will encourage expansion of the roles of the significant others in the scene as well, thus engaging social investigation techniques.

Acting out current events in one's life often arouses emotions that link them with past experiences in one way or another. The astute director capitalizes on this phenomenon and the protagonist unites formative experiences with current ones. The connection of current experiences with older ones happens in narrative therapies as well but the impact that psychodramatic action provides is far more intense and action insight has a greater effect than intellectual insight.

The Sociodramatic Strategy

Sociodrama is concerned with social roles, the role of *the* father, *the* teacher, *the* wife in a specific culture. Protagonists often explore situations that are problematic because the protagonist has found him or herself in an unfamiliar social setting. Perhaps the most common and simplest example is in role training a protagonist for an upcoming event about which the protagonist is anxious. For instance, the protagonist is scheduled for a job interview. It is a job that the protagonist wants very much. The protagonist has never met the interviewer. The director sets the scene of the interview as the protagonist imagines it and has the protagonist begin the interview with an auxiliary employer. After a few initial exchanges, the director calls for a role reversal. The protagonist now becomes the interviewer and the auxiliary is instructed to mirror the protagonist as interviewee. Now the protagonist is in the role of an individual whom the protagonist has never met. The role reversal is a sociometric one, the protagonist relying on his or her understanding of the social role of *the* employer. After a repeat of the initial exchanges, the director interviews the protagonist-in-role-of-employer, asking how well this applicant is doing. Depending upon the answers, the interview can be started if, in the role of employer the protagonist is not satisfied with his performance in the role of applicant, or the interview can be continued with the protagonist in the role of employer asking the most difficult questions that can be imagined. The protagonist then copes with them in the role of applicant.

Other situation in which a director employed a sociometric strategy involved a Caucasian man goes with a Black friend into an all-Black bar; a young woman from a very modest middle class family is invited to a party by a wealthy friend. For both protagonists, the situations generated great anxiety. The sociodramatic work allowed protagonists to experience the unfamiliar roles. It also gave group members an opportunity to enact familiar social roles or explore unknown ones.

Comments on the Uses of These Strategies

Each of the approaches outlined here can be helpful to the protagonist. Each is especially effective under certain conditions. The psychodynamic approach, in my opinion, is a limited one. As an adjunct to other strategies, however, it can be helpful. A good indication for its application is when the protagonist is resistant in the psychodramatic sense. That is, the protagonist finds it difficult or impossible to carry out the director's directions. Dramatizing the internal block to action either resolves it or indicates the direction that the drama should go. I recommend anchoring intrapersonal exploration in time, space, and situation. Otherwise it is difficult to achieve any resolution or movement by the exploring of internal dynamics. The group finds it difficult to stay warmed up or to stay deeply involved during a long intrapersonal psychodramatic sequence.

I have a personal predilection for the strategy that I call psychodramatic. It is a story telling approach to psychodrama. This fits the existential nature of psychodrama and the spontaneity–creativity theory underlying both life and psychodrama.

Psychodrama is modeled after life, Moreno noted, and life consists of one time, place, and situation after another. We tackle the problems of the situation we are in and this activity brings us to and helps form the next. This perspective is a helpful one from which to direct a psychodrama.

My emphasis upon the importance of story telling is supported by Sheldon Kopp (1972), a well-known, highly respected psychotherapist and author, who wrote:

> Each man's identity is an emergent of the myths, ritual, and corporate legends of his culture, compounded with the epic of his own personal history. In either case, it is the compelling power of the storytelling that distinguishes men from beasts. The paradoxical interstice of vulnerability, which makes a man most human rests on his knowing who he is right now, because he can remember who he has been, and because he knows who he hopes to become. All this comes from of the wonder of his being able to tell his tale
>
> *(p. 14)*

Kopp adds a quote from Eli Wiesel: "God made man because he loves stories."

The other strategies are easily incorporated into the story telling mode which also facilitates psychodramatic psychotherapy. Once the protagonist has enacted a an event that resulted in a loss of emotional equilibrium, an emotional reparative psychodramatic experience is often apparent. The protagonist is allowed to express anger at teacher who has unjustly accused the protagonist as a student of cheating. The parent who has unfairly criticized or punished a child can be forced to confront the unjust behavior. The child who was inadequately nurtured can be comforted by a psychodramatic mother or father. Many psychodramas follow a format of a scene of "this is how it actually happened" by a scene of "this is how it *should* have happened."

A psychodrama which tells the protagonist's story communicates more deeply to the members of the group, both those who take auxiliary roles and those who simply witness, representing world opinion as Moreno once described the audience. The protagonist's story communicates to deeper levels of us, stirs us nearer the central parts of ourselves, than does psychodynamic or sociometric material. Telling the story also fits with the fact that psychodrama is above all an art form. Psychodrama literally makes the protagonist the hero or heroine of his or her own life. It reveals both the uniqueness of the protagonist and his or her commonness with others, and in sharing the other members of the group have a chance to experience their respective likenesses and differences. Storytelling is the approach which stands to make the best use of infinitely rich potentials of psychodrama.

Note

1 Certification was originally offered only by the Moreno Institute. After Moreno's death, a certification board, The American Board of Certification in Psychodrama,

Sociometry and Group Psychotherapy was established by the American Society for Group Psychotherapy and Psychodrama. Training requirements for the Certified Practitioner certificate include 780 hours of training with a certified trainer. There are additional requirements for certification.

References

Abraham, A. (1972). Death and psychodrama. *Group Psychotherapy & Psychodrama*, 25, 84–92.

American Psychiatric Association (2015). *Diagnostic and Statistical Manual of Mental Disorders*. Arlington, VA: American Psychiatric Association Publishing.

Barbour, A. (1992). Purpose and strategy behind the magic shop. *Group Psychotherapy, Psychodrama & Sociometry*, 45, 91–101.

Becker, E. (1973). *The Denial of Death*. New York: The Free Press.

Compernolle, T. (1981). J. L. Moreno: An unrecognized pioneer of family therapy. *Family Process*, 20, 331–335.

Enneis, J. (1943). The hypnodramatic technique. *Group Psychotherapy*, 3, 11–54.

Garcia, A. (n.d.) The walk and talk: What it is and how to do it. www.psychodramatraining.com/article2.htm. Accessed March 3, 2015.

Greenberg, I. A. (1977). *Group Hypnotherapy and Hypnodrama*. Chicago, IL: Nelson-Hall.

Haskell, M. R. (1957). Psychodramatic role training in preparation for release on parole. *Group Psychotherapy*, 10, 51–59.

Haskell, M. R. (1959). Role training and job placement of adolescent delinquents: The Berkshire Farm after-care program. *Group Psychotherapy*, 12, 250–257.

Haskell, R. J. & Larr, A. L. (1974). Psychodramatic role training with stutterers. *Group Psychotherapy & Psychodrama*, 27, 30–36.

Hudgens, M. K. (2002). *Experiential Treatment for PTSD: The Therapeutic Spiral Model*. New York: Springer.

Kopp, S. (1972). *If You Meet the Buddah on the Road, Kill Him*. Palo Alto, CA: Science and Behavior Books.

Marineau, R. (1989). *Jacob Levy Moreno, 1889–1974*. New York: Routledge.

Moreno, J. D. (2014). *Impromptu Man*. New York: Bellvue Literary Press.

Moreno, J. L. (1939). Psychodramatic shock therapy: A sociometric approach to the problems of mental disorders. *Sociometry*, 2, 1–30.

Moreno, J. L. (1946a). Psychodrama and group psychotherapy. *Sociometry*, 9, 249–253.

Moreno, J. L. (1946b). *Psychodrama, First Volume*. Beacon, NY: Beacon House.

Moreno, J. L. (1950). Hypnodrama and psychodrama. *Group Psychotherapy*, 3, 1–10.

Moreno, J. L. (1951). Fragments from the psychodrama of a dream. *Group Psychotherapy*, 3, 344–365.

Moreno, J. L. (1952). Psychodramatic production techniques. *Group Psychotherapy*, 4, 243–273.

Moreno, J. L. (1953a). Preludes of the sociometric movement. In J. L. Moreno (Ed.). *Who Shall Survive?*. Beacon, NY: Beacon House. xiii–cviii.

Moreno, J. L. (1953b). *Who Shall Survive?* Beacon, NY: Beacon House.

Moreno, J. L. (1954). Psychodramatic frustration test. *Group Psychotherapy*, 6, 137–167.

Moreno, J. L. (1959). Psychodrama of a dream. In J. H. Masserman & J. L. Moreno (Eds.). *Progress in Psychotherapy*. New York: Grune & Stratton. 193–211.

Moreno, J. L. (1966). Psychodrama of a marriage; a motion picture. *Group Psychotherapy*, 1966, 49–93.

Moreno, J. L. (1973). Notes on indications and contra-indications for acting out in psychodrama. *Group Psychotherapy & Psychodrama*, 26, 23–24.
Moreno, J. L. & Schwartz, M. (1948). Psychodrama combined with insulin in the treatment of psychosis. *Psychiatric Quarterly*, 22, 621–633.
Moreno, Z. T. (1965). Psychodramatic rules, techniques and adjunctive methods. *Group Psychotherapy*, 18, 73–86.
Moreno, Z. T. (1991). Time, space, reality and the family: Psychodrama with a blended (reconstituted) family. In M. Karp & P. Holmes (Eds.). *Psychodrama, Inspiration and Technique*. London: Routledge. 53–74.
Nolte, J. (2008). Protagonist without a problem. In *The Psychodrama Papers*. Lulu.com.
Nolte, J., Weistart, J. & Wyatt, J. (1977). Psychodramatic production of dreams. *Group Psychotherapy, Psychodrama, & Sociometry*, 30, 37–48.
Rackow, L. L. (1951). Modified insulin psychodrama and rehabilitation techniques in the treatment of anxiety and tension states. *Group Psychotherapy*, 4, 214–222.
Seabourne, B. (1963). The action sociogram. *Group Psychotherapy*, 16, 145–155.
Siroka, R. & Schloss, G. (1968). The death scene in psychodrama. *Group Psychotherapy*, 21, 202–205.
Yablonsky, L. (1954). Notes on psychodramatic methods and procedures: Future projection technique. *Group Psychotherapy*, 7, 303–306.

5

PROTAGONISTS DESCRIBE THEIR DRAMAS

As I was preparing to write a book about the practice of psychodrama, the thought occurred to me to invite people who had been engaged in psychodrama and had been protagonists a number of times to write about their most valuable psychodramatic experiences. I invited about 20 people who were currently attending the psychodrama training workshops that I have been conducting with Kätlin Larimer for a number of years to write a description of an important psychodrama in which they had been the protagonist. The request was that the contributor would describe a psychodrama that had made a difference in his or her life. I reserved the right to edit the description with the contributor's approval of the final form. All but one of the people that I approached accepted the invitation. Most expressed some degree of enthusiasm for the project. I was surprised then when only four people completed the project. One person after another informed me that they had looked forward to the assignment but when they sat down to write, they found it impossible to accomplish. Some could not identify which drama to write about. Others knew the drama but found that they could recall very little of what happened in it. All were most apologetic and several have promised to complete the assignment. Two of the people who completed the task did so very quickly. Both their dramas were on dreams.

Moreno contended that when we are fully warmed up to the spontaneity state and are totally in the moment, there is little mental energy left to record the events of that moment. The observer part of the self has disappeared. I think that my project was an unwitting experiment that may have added some confirmation to this idea. I have debated with myself about whether or not to include this chapter but decided to honor those who gave me their gifts, these accounts of their personal psychodramas.

Following are four accounts by protagonists of seven psychodramas as they recalled them, plus another psychodrama in which the writer was an auxiliary.

Protagonist One

(The first writer jumped on my request for an account of a psychodrama with great enthusiasm. However, she was not satisfied with just describing one psychodrama. She found herself recounting a psychodrama journey that encompassed five dramas, in four of which she was protagonist and in the fifth she was the major auxiliary ego.

You might say that she did not follow my instructions. I say that I did not give her the right instructions. I am including her whole contribution because it is such a beautiful example of psychodrama as a method of personal growth. Following is her account.)

I recall a series of dramas that allowed me to first confront and then forgive my parents. These stories helped me identify the abuse and neglect I experienced as well as come to understand how my parents became the people they were. The biggest benefit was me knowing who I was and exploring who I could become.

Drama One

An early drama dealt with my father's controlling, compulsive, and unpredictable behaviors. I started by walking in a circle with the director around "my" life-stage mentioning examples. Certain doors had to be open or shut, lights off or on, the dinner table set with specific items. The director and auxiliaries helped recreate a scene when I was eight or nine years old. My father threw me across the room simply because I left a butter wrapper on the couch arm. I spun through the air like a pinwheel, twisting towards the sliding glass door sliding door. I dropped right before the door; my father stormed away. I think I ran into the woods to hide. My mother came home and no-one shared what dad had done. It was like nothing had happened.

The director had me pick a person to play my eight-year-old self. As I watched from the side, auxiliaries performed the scene. Then the director instructed the me-as-adult to confront dad and take care of my little self. This was the first drama that altered my perception of my family. There was a reason I avoided spending any time with my parents. My father was mentally ill and an alcoholic and my mother in deep denial that led to neglect. I had been abused and it was a secret—I had to be a "good" girl. This was not a loving, healthy family. I wasn't crazy for being scared and enraged. And the abuse was still going on.

Drama Two

The warm up to the next drama included three quick stories and a vignette. I was telling my therapist about dad recently taking me to his local bar, drinking too much and talking about me like I was his lover to the guys there. I went to the bar bathroom and almost passed out from anxiety. Once again upon returning to my parents' house, I acted like nothing happened. My therapist told me that this was sexual abuse, didn't I understand that this was totally inappropriate?

Next, I shared that during a visit home, I told my mom about the abuse with my sisters present. I learned mom had broken my confidence and told my dad that I believed he abused me. I avoided seeing my parents for months. In a vignette scene, I finally visited my parents for my birthday. My drunk father wanted to talk to me alone in his bedroom of all places. He said, "I did not say those things in the bar." For the first time in my life I confronted him, "You *did* do that. I am your daughter. It's not right, the way you treated me!" He broke down and cried, "I would never do anything to hurt you. I am sorry." I sat next to him and told him that I forgave him. Yet, when we went out to fancy dinner, dad was verbally abusive to my mom and me. He was loud and people noticed. Again, I wanted to run away—I was scared.

I paused in the scene—turning, I reached out to the director. Overwhelmed with fear, I suddenly collapsed—my knees gave way. The director helped me fall to the floor. The director instructed auxiliaries to place a bed under me—I was whimpering. The director sat down close to me but not touching and asked, "How old are you?" I shared in a tiny voice, "Very little, 4 or so." Director—"What is happening?" I said, "I hear my father's footsteps approaching down the hall. He burst into my bedroom and sees toys strewn across the floor. He pushes me over the bed and is beating me on my legs. Then storms out." The director gently pushed the middle of my back, gently encouraging me to let go—let it out—I sobbed with tears.

Once I quieted, the director held me and gently brought me back to my adult self asking what I needed to do. I said, "I am very angry. I just want my dad out of my life." I was invited to push my "auxiliary" father out of my life multiple times with force off the stage. In role reversals, playing my father, he kept coming back—he wasn't going to let me be free. The director coached me to use my body and voice. Each time, I became more aware of my strength. I finally screamed in a deep, bold voice, "Get out of my life—stay out!" And my father did stay off the stage. In a quiet conversation with the director, I confirmed there was something very wrong with my father, and I began to wonder what happened to him as a child. I realized I did not have to be haunted by my father's behavior or be afraid of him. I also gained clarity that while my father was sexually inappropriate verbally, there was no memory of actual physical sexual abuse which had haunted me for many years.

Drama Three

In this drama, I confronted my mother about not protecting me from my father's abuse. Starting, I pulled up everyone in my family and described their relationship with me completing many short role reversals. I presented my mother as the perfect mother, community activist, and church leader. I gave a long list of good things she had done. I perceived her as an angel—as untouchable. How could I confront her as neglectful when she had done so much for others? The director told me to let her hear the truth, to tell her what she had done, how I really knew her. I couldn't do it. Double auxiliaries jumped up yelling what I felt, but I froze. I sensed I was going to lose my mind sharing quietly, "I'm afraid I will step over the line and go crazy." The director drew an imaginary line across the floor between me and the auxiliary playing mom. He said, "Step over the line. You can go crazy. I will be here and bring you back." I said, "Really?" and hesitated. He replied, "Yes, go ahead step over the line." He commanded, "TELL her the truth," in a bold voice. Suddenly free, I pounced, I screamed, I cursed at her. It did not matter why, at that point, she did what she did. It felt critical that I had witnesses to what really happened: the secrets, the control, the neglect, the lack of protection, the silly religious rules, mom never leaving an abusive, sick husband. The director asked me several times, "Is there more? What else?" I would do more. I smacked a bataka on a chair! I cursed—I roared, "You abandoned me to the worse abuse. You insist on me being a good girl. You ignore all that is happening—when I was little and even now! You are a horrible mother!" Finally, no more to confront, the director said, "Done?" With a little grin, I revealed, "Yes—that was great!" The director held out his hand and showed me where the line between sane and crazy was on the stage. I took a firm hold as I strongly stepped back across the line feeling clear and strong.

Next, the director had me reverse roles with my mother and, using multiple chairs, I peeled back the layers of who my mother was. The director interviewed my mother with me in her role. She expressed jealousy of me because of my close relationship with her father. My mom wanted to know if I wanted to be with my father because I dated much older men. She blamed me for his sexual inappropriateness. I confronted her saying none of that was true and more evidence that she was in denial of his mental illness and her own neglect. Sitting in the next chair back, my mother revealed that my grandmother had told her God would help her save my dad. Going deeper still in the next chair back, my mother admitted how sick my father was and that she had no idea what to do—but she was afraid if she left him he would die—he was so dependent on her.

The drama helped me realize that my father wanted me to be his substitute wife and my mother wanted me to be a pure, good, little girl. No wonder I felt crazy and confused. Yet, I did not have to be scared that I would become my parents. I could create a self that was beyond my family history.

Dramas Four and Five

The next two psychodramas back to back, at a training workshop, together had a powerful effect. I was protagonist in one and an important auxiliary in the other. The first re-enacted an event where my father made my sister and me choose between breaking dishes or being spanked because we left dishes outside to feed the cats and did not bring them back into the house. It was a horrible scene. I had to watch my sister being whipped as she tried to escape the smacks. In shame and fear, I picked breaking the dishes. My mom sat with her hand tightly over her mouth not intervening. With role reversals, I created a father monster—a crusted, hunkering, crablike figure. I confronted him and he smothered me. I realized he was actually a pathetic creature clinging to me. I dragged the monster to the toilet and flushed him down the drain out of my life—he was dead. I felt immense freedom and claimed my own life with a soliloquy dancing across the stage describing who my real self was—a free spirit with her own choices—her own way of living. Quieting, I wondered out loud if my dad was slowly committing suicide with alcohol because he regretted his behaviors so much, ones that he seemed unable to control. An intense sensation of compassion for his suffering flooded over me. I remained in a very altered state.

That evening, another group member portrayed a drama and picked me to play her younger, sensual self who lost a love. She was betrayed. It was probably one of the most accurate auxiliary roles I ever played. By ridding myself of my father's hold over me, I could emerge. There was a powerful bond between the protagonist and myself. The role brought me back into the world and also helped the protagonist heal. It gave me a star role emerging from my ongoing victim role. It was quite the gift, those two dramas back to back. This week long session was the turning point, where I became more of a trainee and less of a client. I could witness dramas instead of falling into the story.

Conclusion

My dramas and bearing witness to others' dramas helped me emerge into my true self. I could finally make some sense of my father's mental illness and inappropriate attachment, that was sexual, obsessive, controlling, and dependent—combined with his deep regret for hurting me. I accepted that my mom was lost too—just trying to get through day-to-day. My mantra evolved—I could create who I wanted to be. I did not have to confront or "get back" at my folks or be them. They were suffering enough—I did not need to add to it. I became more tender and compassionate towards them, yet, better at taking care of myself.

I was on my own path. I was able to settle into my life and be more present, more spontaneous, and make wiser choices. I moved to another city and left behind my old self, to begin anew. I have had an incredible career of helping others, wonderful friends, married a great guy and had a son—raising him very differently. My husband even joined me in psychodrama training. While I am still working to be more me, I am living a full and very, present life.

Protagonist Two

(As the writer notes, this drama took place during a training workshop. The trainer supervisor was quite active in coaching the student director who had never directed a dream psychodrama and was not familiar with the structure that J. L. Moreno had established for dramatizing dreams.)

This drama occurs at a psychodrama training workshop. It's day three and a late afternoon session. There are about eight of us in the room, one of the trainers and a few friends I know from other workshops.

I had these constant nightmares, as many as five out of seven nights a week, most weeks. It was always the same, some kind of fight with my brother. I can be in a store shopping or be eating somewhere and he just shows up. Punching me, grabbing me mostly, like when we were kids, he was much larger than me and picked on me often. I fight back and then I awake agitated upset and can't go back to sleep. I have to say that the drama is still somewhat of a blur I may miss parts of what happened. So I will just tell it as I best I now recall it, a few years later.

I offer to be the protagonist for this session and pick another group member to be the director:

P: I had another nightmare last night. I have them almost every night now for the last three years or so. It's about my older brother. You know something about him from other dramas I have done. In the dream he shows up bullying me, pushing and grabbing. *(I can feel myself starting to get upset, my hands are starting to sweat and I feel this pit in my stomach and I am tensing up. I am starting to picture some of the dreams in my mind.)*

DIRECTOR: Well instead of telling us, show us. Let's begin by you showing us how you go to bed.

I go through the motions of getting ready for bed and get into bed, represented by a mattress on the floor.

DIRECTOR: Lie down and go to sleep like you usually do. Soliloquize your thoughts as you to sleep.

I lie down on the bed to my right. I pull the cover up to my neck and lie on my side like I always do and close my eyes. I speak some thoughts out loud. I may have said, "I hope I don't have that dream tonight." The director tells me to go to sleep and let the time pass until the dream starts and then signal that I am dreaming. After a while I signal.

DIRECTOR: Let yourself have the dream.

I have no idea how much time passes. It feels like at least five minutes or more. I am relaxing and the prior agitation is starting to go away. It's very quiet I can't feel anyone else in the room … Here comes the dream. Here I have to say I am not sure how much of this I remember. I do know I was talking to someone and all of a sudden my brother appears and says something like "Hey asshole" and pushes me. I push back. He grabs me behind my neck and pulls me towards him. I feel myself breathing hard.

DIRECTOR: You are in the dream?

ME: Yes. Yes.

DIRECTOR: Ok. Get up now and show us what is happening. How does the dream begin? What is the first scene?

I get up. I feel agitated my arms are tense (*In fact as I write this I feel agitated and my arms are tense.*) I notice that the room seems darker, somebody turned out the big light there is only a corner light.

DIRECTOR: Where are you?

ME: I am in this bar.

DIRECTOR: Ok. Set the scene.

ME: There is this bar right here. There are chairs right over here. There's a TV on the wall here, some people over there, and I am talking to this guy.

DIRECTOR: Who is this person you are talking to?

Me I don't know. I think just some guy.

DIRECTOR: Pick him out for us from the group.

(*I picked someone that kind of reminded me of him.*)

DIRECTOR: Role reverse with him. (*To me reversed into his role.*) What are you saying to this guy?

(*I can't remember what he or I was saying now but whatever it was I said it and then reversed with him. I also am pretty warmed up. I see someone in our group who has played my brother before and I see him as my brother as I am reversing back into myself.*)

DIRECTOR: Is your brother here yet?

ME: Not yet but I see him. (*I point to the man in our group who has played my older brother before.*)

DIRECTOR: Reverse roles with your brother and tells us who you are.

ME (*REVERSED AS MY BROTHER*): I am [Protagonist's] older brother I am 6'3" 195 great shape good looking.

DIRECTOR: How do you feel about your brother here?

ME (*STILL REVERSED AS MY BROTHER*): He thinks he's so smart and shit. I don't like him, never really did.

DIRECTOR: Show us what you do to your brother.

ME (*STILL REVERSED AS BROTHER*): Hey ASSHOLE! (*I show how I push him and then grab him behind the neck.*)

DIRECTOR: Reverse back. Is there anyone else in this scene?

ME: No just some people sitting over there drinking and talking—it's a bar you know.

DIRECTOR: (*To group members*) Some of you go sit over there.

They do and start to talk very softly and pretend to drink.

DIRECTOR: (*To me*) Start to talk to the person at the bar and older brother, you come in and do what you do.

The scene is acted out. The auxiliary as my brother says "Hey ASSHOLE!" comes up and pushes me. I push back. He grabs me behind the neck and pulls me towards him. I push hard back. It's a real struggle. The auxiliary is a big guy like my brother. I don't hold back and neither does he.

ME: Then I wake up

DIRECTOR: Soliloquize.

ME: Fuck I hate this! I hate him! I wish he would just leave me alone. Fuck this … (*I start to tear up and cry.*) I can't take this anymore. I don't even want to go to sleep. I drink a half a bottle of wine to just get the courage some nights to go to sleep. *(At this point I still feel as I did in the dream, I feel mad . angry. I can still see my brother sitting over there and yes, he looks like my brother, not himself.*)

There seems to be a few minutes that go by, I am staring at the auxiliary older brother. I think I am settling down but I really can't remember … I don't know what happens exactly after this, I am pretty upset, crying I think. I think the director has us strike the scene. I think he had me tell my brother to fuck off and leave, I do and my brother leaves the room. Some time during this the lights are turned up.

DIRECTOR: Now the next thing we are going to do is to change this dream. You obviously don't want it as you have dreamed it. You can change anything and everything that you want. The first scene of the original dream is in a bar. Do you want to change that?

ME: Well it's the same bar. But instead of a guy, there is this really pretty blond here I am talking to. There are still people over there and this other really pretty girl walks up to me and says "hi." They remind me of two girls I used to hang out with. One is a really hot blond or was 20 years ago and the other is a pretty brown-haired girl. Both are pretty free spirits we had some pretty fun times together for over a year or so.

The director has me pick out auxiliaries to be the girls. I reverse roles with each of them and describe them in the role reversal. Then we talk and are getting along great. Then I say:

ME: Hey, I've got an idea. Why don't we go back to my place. I've got a hot tub and I will make us something to eat.

DIRECTOR: Reverse roles with the blonde.

ME-AS-THE-BLONDE: Oh, do you cook?

ME: No. I don't cook. I create dishes.

Then we act out going back to my place. I show them around my house which is pretty neat, and then we get in the hot tub together.

The director then has me set up the first scene, my bedroom here. "This time I want you to go back to sleep and you are going to have this new dream." I lay down, I think somebody turned out the big light. Minutes go by as I go back to my simulated sleep.

DIRECTOR: Are you dreaming now?

ME: Yes.

DIRECTOR: OK. Have the full dream, everything, meeting the girls, leaving the bar, the hot tub, the whole night everything that happens. Take your time, all the time you need. Feel it all and when it is morning and you are in bed waking up from your sleep, wake up slowly and sit up in bed.

I have my wonderful dream, all of it, I feel relaxed, so relaxed. I have some conception of time so it is like 10 minutes or so go by. I am in no hurry to wake, but it starts to feel like morning and my dream has already come to an end. And I wake up and sit up in bed. I feel a little sleepy still and relaxed.

DIRECTOR: How was that?

ME: Great, I feel really relaxed right now.

DIRECTOR: Next time you start to have that bad dream or you are worried about that bad dream, remember the good dream.

After that the group members shared with me. I don't recall exactly what was said. Some people talked about bad dreams they have had, some about good dreams, some about bullies and one I remember was about an old girlfriend. Since that drama I have not had the nightmares of my brother. I feel like I may have had one or two start but were stopped. I did have one that I can remember, and remember waking up mad at myself that I did not stop it. But I must say that the nightly nightmares are gone. My sleep is so, so, so much better. I don't wake up in a sweat. The drama has helped literally change my life and for that I thank the group who was there that night to help me. The drama helped me change my life and the way I think about sleep and how I sleep.

Protagonist Three

This is my memory of the psychodrama about my mother's death. She had been ill for less than 90 days since her first symptom of a neurological problem. The only available diagnostic test in 1971 was a pneumoencephalogram in which they inject air in the spine and then x-ray the brain so the area between the skull and the brain is outlined. It diagnoses tumors on the surface of the brain. My mother's test had come back negative. The neurologist was at a loss. We had been trying to talk my father into taking her to the Mayo Clinic to try to determine what was going on. We were also planning on moving her to a care facility because she could not walk and was incontinent and Dad could no longer take care of her. Then I got a telephone call, when I was waiting to be seated at an old hotel dining room in Omaha where the Reuben Sandwich was invented. My husband and I immediately drove to Lincoln and went directly to the hospital. Dad was there and was an emotional basket case. He just could not handle the situation.

I don't remember quite how the drama got started or even why I chose that moment to re-visit my mother's death. The first scene may have been the telephone call from my Dad or probably my brother calling me to tell me that she had lapsed into a coma and had been taken to the hospital.

The next scene that I remember is my father, my brother, and I checking mom into the hospital. She had lapsed into a coma at home very unexpectedly. It was the day we were moving her to the care facility. Then my brother, his wife, me, my husband and Dad all waited for the neurologist to give us a report. He eventually came into the waiting lounge and gave us the news. For the first time he felt he had a diagnosis: She had a very deep brain tumor, he told us, and probably had about 12 hours to live.

It was a total shock. The neurologist was really just leaving us high and dry, completely helpless. There was nothing he could do, nothing that could be done. Mother was going to die and probably within 12 hours. I was stunned.

The director instructed me express everything that I wanted to say to the neurologist but had been unable to say at the time. I screamed at him. I swore at him. I beat him up for not having an answer and for being so utterly clinical and indifferent. He had told me earlier when I asked him if we should try to push her to do things or not, "My time is for the living, not the dying." That was the first time I had heard that he thought she was going to die.

In the next scene in the drama I am alone in her room all night with her. My brother and his wife could not tolerate being in the room with her, watching her die, breathing less and less regularly. Dad could not tolerate it either so I opted to send my husband home with Dad to care for him. The scene involved me sharing my soliloquy and talking to her. My terror and heartbreaks.

Scene 4 is me deciding to go home about 7 a.m. to check on my Dad, to see how he was doing. Mother appeared to be stable so I thought I had plenty of time. Dad was completely collapsed emotionally and my husband didn't really know what to do with him. That scene involved me expressing my feelings of being so alone. Dad was just totally incapable of stepping up. A year later I learned that he had already had dementia for several years but was covering it. My husband was staying with him but really not helpful. My brother just back from Viet Nam was suffering from untreated PTSD and about to lose his most important emotional connection in the world, his mother. Everything was on me. I felt responsible to take care of everybody. Either I lined them all up I think or maybe I just dealt with Dad and My husband about how I needed help. "I cannot do this alone!" I think maybe I was screaming at Dad … "DO SOMETHING!!!!"

Scene 5: I am returning to the hospital. I could not have been gone more than 45 minutes, tops. I walk into mom's room and it is empty. The bed is made. I felt like I must have gotten disoriented and have gone to an empty room, not hers. Just then a nurse walks in and says "your mother died and we have sent her to the morgue". I cannot believe what I am hearing. Another shock.

In that scene I first replayed it as it happened which was that my brother walked in at that point. Then the director then had me go back and redo the scene, only this time I was free to say and do everything that I felt like saying and doing. What I felt like doing was completely destroying the place. I ripped up the bed, threw the entire contents of the room out the door, beat the neurologist to a pulp, then the nurse … all of them.

Finally, after giving voice to all the anger and rage that I felt at the way my mother had been treated and how I had been treated, I collapsed and sobbed. And sobbed. And sobbed. For a long time.

Scene 6: When my tears finally subsided, the director pointed out that in my concern for my Dad, I had not been with Mother when she died. "Let's give you a chance to do that they way you would have wanted."

Instead of leaving the hospital, this time I stayed and was there with her when she died. I held her hand and told her what was on my mind. Then the director had me reverse roles and experience her death.

Protagonist Four

I suffered a recurrent dream that was not pleasant. I would literally die in the dream by drowning. When I say "die" I mean to say that in the dream my physical body was dead. There was a funeral with attendant and attendees. At the same time, I was always aware and could see those who were mourning and those who were not. My recollection is that at the time of the psychodrama, I had experienced this dream every night for 11 years. I would wake up sweating, out of breath and my heart racing. It was always this same dream with a few minor changes. The only nights that I do not recall the dream in those years were the nights where I had drunk myself to sleep and passed out, more or less. The dream was the same, except that the people who attended the funeral would change. In the dream, I would be driving on a bridge where there was water on both sides and as far as you could see in all directions. There were three other people in the car with me. I could only see the face of one and the other two were there, but their faces were out of focus and I could not ever make them out. We would go off the bridge, struggle unsuccessfully to get out of the car and I would eventually drown. I asked many people, "I thought you were not supposed to die in your dreams?" I would get weird answers and looks from Ph.D.s to M.D.s at this inquiry.

I had never heard the term "dream psychodrama" until one day in a psychodrama training workshop, the director was talking about it. I mentioned my dream and was chosen to be the protagonist. This is what occurred in my first and only dream psychodrama, as well as the result of this experience.

The first scene was me going to bed on a night when I had the dream. I went through my usual preparations and got into bed. Then I was asked to soliloquize my thoughts just before going to sleep. Then the director asked me drift off to sleep and to wait until the dream began. He asked if the dream woke me up and I said it did. He directed me to dream the dream again until it woke me up. I did so, suddenly sitting up in bed when the dream woke me up. The director asked, "How does the dream begin?"

The director then had me reenact the scenes of the dream in live action. We began where the dream always did, in the car on the long bridge. We filled the car with people. As is required generally, I was asked to reverse roles with the auxiliaries in the drama, identify them and give some details. The two people in the drama that I could not make out were still vague to me, but the passenger in the back seat on the passenger's side was coming in clear. I won't say the name here, but I did name her and give details about her in the psychodrama. The director asked me to have a bit of a conversation with her while driving, just before the crash into the drink. I started having a physical reaction, similar to the ones that I have each night. I really don't recall what happened next or how I got on the floor but there I was, dead, drowned lying on the floor. People were looking at me just as they do in the dream. I could hear them and see them but it was like they couldn't hear or see me, only my lifeless body. I wanted them to know, "I am right here!" As the drama unfolded and the funeral progressed, a deep, deep sadness came over me. I could not stop weeping. I realized that this dream started about the same time that the woman in the back passenger's seat died of breast cancer and that the dream was about my never having grieved her loss. The rest of the session was spent allowing me the chance to grieve the loss of my dear friend and to comfort her spouse. In real life, I had to be strong for the surviving spouse, because his world was a wreck. Constraining my emotions came out in a weird and unexpected way; I was having a recurring dream about death.

I have not had the dream again and to this day, over ten years later. In addition, my understanding of what may happened after death has been changed. I was no longer afraid of most anything after this drama. Some of the demons that created this fear and kept it around for survival were gone and the fear subsided. I have changed since this drama. I no longer drink alcohol, it will be 12 years in December. I don't need it anymore. The process of allowing me to grieve the loss of this friend, "opened" or "unclogged" a pathway in my body, soul or spirit and effected my mind. I felt a peace that had evaded me for years. I still feel it.

6

BEYOND PSYCHOTHERAPY

In Chapter 1 of this book, I maintained that defining psychodrama as a method of psychotherapy was misleading, and called for a broader, more inclusive one. There is a reason why the definition is important. If psychodrama is defined as psychotherapeutic method, then only licensed mental health professionals are allowed to practice. Yet there are far more occasions for the application of psychodrama techniques and procedures outside the field of psychotherapy than there are within it. This chapter reviews the application of psychodrama in the fields of education, of business and industry, and in the practice of law where trial lawyers have discovered innovative ways of using psychodrama in the preparation for the courtroom.

Role Playing

Moreno first engaged in role playing as a method of teaching children in the *Augarten*, a park in the grounds of the imperial palace, to be spontaneous. As a university student, Moreno walked through the park, forming groups of children for impromptu play.

> It was a kindergarten on a cosmic scale, a creative revolution among children. It was a crusade of children for themselves, for a society of their own age and their own rights. I wanted to give the children the capacity to fight against social stereotypes, against robots, *for* spontaneity and creativity.
>
> *(J. L. Moreno, 1989, p. 37)*

It was during this work with children that Moreno's theories of spontaneity and creativity and took form.

Moreno's regarded his first major venture in adult role playing as the birth of psychodrama. The event took place on April 1, 1921. It was an endeavor to find a king, a leader for Vienna and Austria, then in a state of chaos after World War I. "It was an attempt to treat and purge the audience from a pathological cultural syndrome which all the participants shared. Post war Vienna was seething with revolt. It had no stable government, no emperor, no king, no leader" (J. L. Moreno, 1946b, p. 1). In a theater full of people drawn there by the announcement that the new king would be present at the performance, Moreno appeared on the stage, empty except for a throne-like chair with a gilded crown on it. In what he would later call a spontaneity test, he invited members of the audience to try out for the role. The audience was the jury. No one passed the test and Moreno was taken to task by the newspapers the next morning.

His next venture with adults and role playing, *Das Stegreiftheater*, the Theater of Spontaneity, was more successful. The goal was establishment of a revolutionary theatre that would introduce the concepts of spontaneity and creativity to the whole of society. His fantasy was that the theater would inspire people to greater spontaneity in their lives. The efforts of the players learning how to co-create dramas spontaneously, in the moment, without script or rehearsal, made the theater a laboratory of spontaneity–creativity (J. L. Moreno, 1947b). Two of the major concepts that came out of his research were the spontaneity state and the spontaneity test. Moreno also noted the phenomenon he would later label tele among the players of the spontaneity theater. Sometime during the three-year span of *Das Stegreiftheater*, Moreno then undertook to repair the marital problems of a woman by making use of her role as one of his spontaneity players (more details are in Chapter 8). This event became the prototype for psychodramatic psychotherapy.

Moreno used a number of terms to designate the several methods that he devised, spontaneity testing, spontaneity training, role testing, role training, psychodrama, and sociodrama. All of them are role playing methods, employing one or more psychodramatic techniques such as self presentation, auxiliary egos, and role reversal, and a psychodrama stage. These various methods are sometimes distinguishable only by the goal for which they are being applied. For example, the Search for the King happening that Moreno considered the first psychodrama could also be called role testing. It was at the same time, sociodramatic, exploring the social role of leader, and it was spontaneity training as well. All these procedures are spontaneity methods and are subsets of psychodrama.

Moreno's goal was to turn society, all of humankind, away from its overdependence upon cultural conserves in favor of greater spontaneity in their lives. He had expected that the spontaneously created dramas of the theater of spontaneity would encourage people to live their daily lives with greater spontaneity. However, people had been brought up to rely on established roles and procedures and to distrust their own spontaneity.

> Therefore, when true spontaneity was presented to them in the Stegreiftheater either they suspected it to be well rehearsed and an attempt to fool them, or, if a scene was poorly played they considered that as a sign that spontaneity does not work.
>
> *(J. L. Moreno, 1947b p. 7)*

He saw a tremendous task ahead in the changing of the attitude of the public. This required no less than a cultural revolution. At the same time Moreno also noticed his best actors sometimes repeating themselves in their spontaneity work. Many of them eventually turned away from spontaneity theater and went to the legitimate stage or to Hollywood. "*Faced with this dilemma I turned 'temporarily' to the therapeutic theater, a strategic decision which saved the psychodramatic movement from oblivion*" (J. L. Moreno, 1947b, p. 7, italics in the original). Obviously, he never intended psychodrama to be limited to psychotherapy.

Psychodrama and Education

From the time that he became a tutor of children when he himself was only 16, to his interactions with the children of Vienna in the Augarten, to his psychodramatic work with children at Mt. Sinai Hospital and the Plymouth Institute, to his work at the New York Training School for Girls, Moreno saw the education of children as the starting point for a creative revolution based on the principles of spontaneity. He criticized the approach of how schools operate: "In the formal school and the process of learning and the technique of teaching have no relationship to the things and people with whom the children actually live in their groups outside the school" (Moreno & Jennings, 1936, p. 20). Needs and desires are how young children learn.

> The young child learns through a spontaneous reaching out for the thing it needs. Its learnings are strictly related to acts, its acts and are founded on needs. There is, say, a hunger (a *need* for food) there is *action* to get food, there are *learnings* about food.
>
> *(J. L. Moreno, 1946b, p. 140)*

At a certain age, however, adults inject contents into the child's world prevailing on them to learn poems, songs, facts and the like which have to do with the adult authority's needs, not the child's. The child learns to accept the contents that the authority offers and to mistrust its own creative life. Moreno's prescription of educators: "The reproductive process of learning must move into second place; first emphasis should be given to the productive, spontaneous-creative process of learning. The exercises and training in spontaneity is the chief subject of the future" (J. L. Moreno, 1946b, p. 81).

The publication of *Who Shall Survive?* in 1934 caused a stir, not only in the social sciences, but in the field of education as well. This is not surprising as the book, which detailed Moreno's major research project, took place in a residential school setting. Moreno's preliminary research had also taken place in a school, PS 181, Brooklyn, NY, where, three years before, sociometry had been employed to determine seating arrangements in classrooms. Many of the articles and reports in *Sociometry*, the journal that Moreno established as a medium for exchange of information on sociometry and psychodrama, pertained to schools and education.

Many of the first articles entailed sociometry and social adjustment, leadership, and isolation, reflecting a growing responsibility on the part of schools for promoting good social relationships in students. "One outstanding aim of education is to work and live well with others" (Shoobs, 1947). There was also increased recognition of the relationship between social adjustment and the ability to learn among teachers. In addition to sociometric studies, articles on applications of psychodrama in the classroom also began to appear. Franz (1939) described using both sociometric and psychodramatic techniques to reduce anxiety in students in classes on public speaking. Lippitt (1943) in an article on psychodrama and leadership training described in detail a role training session for the leader of an adult study group. Shoobs (1943, 1944) related the use of psychodrama to deal successfully with a group of truant boys in a Brooklyn school. Zander and Lippitt (1944) used the term "reality practice" to describe teaching a parent-child relationship problem in a sociology class. Kay and Schick (1945) successfully trained interviewers for a study of tensions requiring information from members of three different ethnic groups in a low-income community by role training the prospective interviewers.

In 1947, Moreno started a new journal, initially named *Sociatry,* a term that he had coined and defined as "remedial sociometry" (J. L. Moreno, 1947a). By 1948, enough projects had been conducted that a large part of the 1948 volume of *Sociatry* was devoted to psychodrama and sociodrama in education. The volume was guest edited by Robert Haas and later published as a book, *Psychodrama and Sociodrama in American Education,* (Haas, 1949b). The work consists of 37 articles, grouped into eight sections: one on defining the educational problem; four on projects at different educational levels (elementary, junior high, high school, and college); one on counseling; another on tests and measurements; and a summary section with recommendations for educational practice.

Haas declared that the volume demonstrated that psychodramatic and sociodramatic techniques can make a valuable contribution to education. He recommended that all instructional programs should include human relations work at all grade levels. He also thought that: "Teachers should be increasingly aware of the value of interaction in the learning situation, and experimenting with ways to vary the kinds of interaction in the classroom to intensify the atmosphere for learning" (Haas, 1949b, p. 426). Teachers needed training in sociometric and sociodramatic techniques, he stated, and colleges should establish psychodramatic units to conduct research and train students and teachers. Finally, of course, Haas recommended further research. Haas's recommendations have been largely ignored by the field of education.

There have been, none the less, hundreds of articles on psychodrama and education in both psychodrama and education literature. Applications of psychodramatic techniques and procedures in the field of education were originally called psychodrama, sociodrama, spontaneity testing, spontaneity training, or role training. The term, role playing, was introduced by Kay, a pioneer in introducing psychodrama in education. In 1946, Kay wrote an article on role playing as a teaching aid. She explained in a footnote that "The term 'role-playing situation' is used throughout this article in the same sense as the term 'sociodramatic or psychodramatic situation' by other contributors" (p. 265). Role playing has eventually become the most frequently used term in education as well as in business and industrial settings.

In 2003, Bona Anna, a New Zealand psychodramatist and educator, conducted a herculean review of over 175 such publications. Anna covered both sociometry and psychodrama in her review. She divided it into three eras, the early work up to the publication of *Psychodrama and Sociodrama In American Education* (Haas, 1949b); From the late 1940s and through the 1960s; and the modern era, 1970 to her publication in 2003. Anna reports that she was "struck by the depth of understanding and breadth of vision displayed by those pioneering American educators. The potential of sociometry, sociodrama and psychodrama for educational success was being realised or was implied in their experimental work and research" (p. 71). However, she found that

> The work of more recent decades, however, has not been characterised by the fervour of previous years, and much of the early promise of the sociometric movement has tended to lie dormant, waiting perhaps for modern day educators to take up the mantle *en masse*.
>
> *(p. 71)*

Articles still appear in numerous journals reporting on the use of role playing in the classroom (e.g., Lin, Lake, & Rice, 2008; Simpson & Elias, 2011; Yunker, Orion, & Lernau, 2011; Campbell, 2012; Kassardjian et al., 2013; Gartmeier et al., 2015). Each describes a distinctly different approach to the activity called role playing. None of them refer to Moreno, a Morenean article, or to any author who references Moreno. Role playing is often referred to in an offhand way as if it is a commonplace activity which is universally understood. As Moreno lamented, his methods found widespread acceptance and adoption while the philosophy and theories upon which they were founded were "relegated to the dark corners of library shelves or entirely pushed aside" (J. L. Moreno, 1953a, p. 15. See also Z. T. Moreno, 1967).

An excellent presentation of sociodrama and its many possible applications is Sternberg and Garcia's *Sociodrama: Who's in Your Shoes?* (1989). Most classroom role playing is sociodramatic rather than psychodramatic. That is, the roles that are enacted are social roles rather than psychodramatic or personal ones. In addition to offering a detailed course in directing sociodrama, Sternberg and Garcia provide the theoretical underpinnings of the method. They also put forward suggestions on how sociodrama can be used in teaching history, social studies, languages, literature, psychology, nursing, and more. Another source is *Role Playing in the Curriculum* (2nd ed) by Shaftel and Shaftel (1982).

Haas's recommendations are still worthy after more than 70 years. There is much in sociometry, psychodrama, sociodrama, and group psychotherapy, both theoretical and methodological, from which the field of education could greatly profit. Shearon and Shearon (1973) suggest that knowledge and the use of the concepts of warm up, spontaneity and spontaneity training, creativity, tele, sociometry, social atom, and role reversal "could revolutionize the entire school setting …" (p. 49).

Psychodrama in Business and Industry

The introduction of sociometry via *Who Shall Survive?* in 1934 had an impact in industry as it did in the field of education. Industry had done exceedingly well in fulfilling its function of producing material goods. But industry has another important function, to make factory work meaningful and to produce human satisfactions for workers. It had been slow to recognize this responsibility. Social science was even slower in generating experimental results in this respect that industry could use. One idea that caught the attention of industrial psychologists was the sociometric notion of a hidden social structure functioning under the formal structure of the organization (Rogers, 1946). Jacobs (1945) contributed an early article describing sociometric practice in one department of the company where he worked, and many more publications followed in *Sociometry* and other journals.

Psychodrama in the form of role training as a means of training the employees of a company or organization caught on to an even greater extent than did sociometry. Perhaps Lippitt's (1943) article on leadership training was one of the first. By 1953, psychologist Norman R. F. Maier wrote,

> Since Moreno developed the method of role playing, first as a training procedure and later as a therapeutic technique, its potentialities are becoming more and more apparent. A great variety of applications and procedures have been developed so that practically every form of social adjustment has been explored to some degree.
>
> *(1953, p. 31)*

Maier was a well-known psychologist at the University of Michigan. After a successful career as an experimental psychologist, he turned to the experimental study of human factors in business and industry around 1945. Maier wrote several books (1952, 1955a, 1955b, 1962, 1965, 1975; Maier, Solem, & Maier, 1957) and numerous papers on psychology in industry. His first book, *Principles of Human Relations* (1952) featured two chapters on role playing as a training method, and he continued to endorse it throughout his career, his 1975 book entitled *Role Play Technique: Handbook for Management and Leadership Practice.*

Maier (1952) discussed other training methods and pointed out that the methods chosen for a training task had to be appropriate for the objective of the training. He discussed a number of objectives for which he believed role training was uniquely fitted. Role training helps supervisors realize that they need training and "permits each person to learn what he needs most" (p. 91). It helps correct the gap between knowing and doing better than methods like lecturing and reading. Role training is especially effective in developing skills in recognizing the feelings of others, learning to listen and accept the feelings of others as genuine instead of criticizing, arguing, and rejecting. Changing attitudes toward others, toward oneself, or toward the job can also be accomplished by the method. Another advantage of the method is that "Role playing carries the training into action. This is actually one of the major benefits ..." (p. 99). Here Maier is recognizing the increase in spontaneity of participants in role playing even though he doesn't use the word spontaneity. Role playing, Maier says, "may serve the same function for human relations training as clinical experience serves the young doctor of medicine" (p. 99).

Maier considered role training to be superior to on-the-job training. The advantage, he claimed, is that people are less inhibited in role playing and more likely to express what they feel.

> This amounts to magnifying behavior effects and making them more apparent and less likely to go unnoticed. After a person has seen the magnified reactions in the roles played he is more likely to recognize them in real-live situations ere people tend to hide their hostilities, their dislikes, or their fears.
>
> *(p. 100)*

Delbert Miller (1951) wrote "Business administrators are beginning to see references to role playing in such magazines as *Fortune, Business Week*, and *Personnel.* They are reading about the use of role playing in the supervisory training programs of many highly regarded companies" (p. 48). According to Miller, of the University of Washington, there was great excitement among leaders in business, education, government, and agriculture in the Pacific Northwest about role playing. Even the Boeing Aircraft Company had introduced a series of training programs using role playing techniques. Miller wrote that role playing was appearing in Family Life meetings and in the classrooms of both elementary schools and colleges, and adults were being introduced to role playing through the Adult Education Center of the University of Washington. Even PTA members were coming home with reports of role playing events.

Miller, who had first experienced demonstrations of role playing at Moreno's Sociometric Institute in 1947, was responding to numerous requests for presentations of the method from business associations, government administrators, and supervisors. They wanted to see what can be done with it in business and government. Miller described three applications of role playing in industry and government: as a conference technique for problem solving; a technique for employment selection; and a training method for employees and supervisors.

The introduction of role training into industry was markedly stimulated by the National Training Laboratories, an organization founded by Kurt Lewin in 1947. Lewin was an academic psychologist associated with the Gestalt school of psychology who fled Nazi Germany in 1933. A mutual acquaintance, Alfred Marrow, introduced Lewin and Moreno, in 1935. Lewin had become interested in social psychology, probably as a result of the rise of Nazism, and was aware of Moreno's sociometry, having read *Who Shall Survive?* He and Moreno had several meetings during which he explored Moreno's ideas. Lewin then sent students to the Psychodrama Institute for training in Morenean methods. Lewin, with several of his students, founded the National Training Laboratories for Group Development in 1947. Although Lewin died before the National Training Laboratories became active, the organization continued under the leadership of Kenneth Benne, Leland Bradford and Ronald Lippitt, all of whom had trained with Moreno. The NTL Institute, as it is known today, was interested in organization development from its earliest days. Role training, often called role playing, was one of the methods that NTL consultants demonstrated and recommended (Miller, 1951).

Psychologist John R. P. French, Jr. was a Lewin student and another early contributor to industrial psychology and organizational development. He published an account of role training foremen at Harwood Manufacturing Corporation, a sewing plant that employed 650 workers in 1945. French stated that compared to methods such as reading, lectures, conferences and discussion, role playing is distinctively different:

> It is a dramatic play-like activity on an *irreal* plane. Paradoxically, it is also very concrete and *realistic*-probably as close as possible to actual job performance … [and] it stimulates participation, involvement, and identification in such a way as to bring out the deeper *emotional* aspects of interpersonal relations.
>
> *(1945, p. 183)*

French found a number of virtues of role training. It solved the problem of transfer of training and provides an excellent bridge from talking about interpersonal relations to actually handling them (p. 421). It quickly helps the trainer identify the needs of the trainee, and permits immediate coaching "whereas on-the-job training usually necessitates a longer gap between performance on the one hand and reward and punishment on the other hand" (p. 183). The method is flexible and is an effective way of countering rigidity and resistance to change.

French thought role training was particularly valuable for the training of foremen who are workers in some respects and members of management in others. This puts them in particularly vulnerable position when there is conflict between management and employees, a common situation. "Thus the problems of position and status are unusually acute for him, and role-playing seems particularly adapted to handling such inter-personal problems" (p. 187). It helps the supervisor trainee become sensitive to the feelings of the workers they oversee when they get to play the role of worker in role training exercises.

The several early contributors to role playing in business and industry are characteristic of literature on the subject which grew exponentially through the 1960's. Role training in industry, is no longer a novelty. It continues to be practiced in a variety of ways by trainers and organizational development consultants. However, it has almost entirely lost its connection with psychodrama and J. L. Moreno. It is likely that few practitioners of role playing in the field are aware of the provenance of the methods they are using or of the benefits that understanding psychodramatic techniques might have for their work.

Psychodrama and Trial Lawyers

When Gerry Spence decided to start his Trial Lawyers College (TLC), he arranged for it to begin with a psychodrama experience. Spence, famed lawyer and certainly one of the most successful, had long aspired to teach young lawyers the trial skills that had made him uniquely successful. Encouraged in this endeavor by his close friends, he remodeled buildings on his ranch near Dubois, Wyoming, to serve as dormitory and classrooms, and, in the summer of 1994, established the College. The first class consisted of 48 trial lawyer students, with a dozen of Spence's veteran colleagues as instructors. The event occupied the whole month of August.

It is significant to note that Spence was interested in sharing his singular trial skills only with civil plaintiff lawyers and criminal defense lawyers. These lawyers have people for clients. Lawyers who represented insurance companies or corporations, as well as prosecutors were not admitted to the Trial Lawyers College. Insurance company and corporation lawyers always have much greater resources to draw on, and prosecutors have all the resources of government available to them. The lawyers representing people are always at some degree of disadvantage.

Spence had discovered psychodrama through his friend and colleague, John Ackerman, then Dean of the National College of Criminal Defense, an organization that provided post-graduate training events for inexperienced trial lawyers. Ackerman had sought a means for teaching lawyers to be more creative. Psychodrama had been suggested as a means to do that and the National College of Criminal Defense had presented a series of programs entitled "The Criminal Trial: A Psychodramatic Analysis," but what were actually group centered, 2½ day psychodrama workshops. Spence had been a part of both the planning and the initial presentation. Don Clarkson, an experienced psychodramatist, had directed for those programs.

Spence was convinced that the ability to accurately read one's emotions and incorporate them into one's actions as well as sensitivity to others' feelings, emotional intelligence, was essential to a trial lawyer's success in the charged intensity of the courtroom. He was equally certain that psychodrama was the best way of increasing that skill. He scheduled three days of personal growth psychodrama to begin and two days to end the 30 day program of the Trial Lawyers College. He engaged Don Clarkson and me to direct the psychodrama.

Not knowing about the positive reception that the psychodrama programs of N.C.C.D. had received, I arrived at Spence's Thunderhead Ranch with some anxiety about how trial lawyers would respond to psychodrama. I could imagine great resistance and even a mutiny ("We came here to learn about trial lawyer skills, not do this personal stuff!"). To my surprise, the lawyers seemed more open to psychodrama than the average mental health professional. The first three days went very quickly. We did a number of meaningful personal psychodramas.

Expanding the Use of Psychodrama

I arrived at the first TLC in 1994, knowing nothing about the objectives of the College or how they were to be taught. I learned that the program involved training in a number of different skills which a trial lawyer needs to conduct a trial. If skills are being taught, I thought, role training might be an effective way to teach them. I informed Spence that psychodrama might have more to offer TLC than just the personal growth and development. He was open to the suggestion and invited me to stay. I could not stay but agreed to come back next year prepared to spend more time at the College and contribute to the program.

Clarkson and I conducted the three days of personal psychodrama and then left the ranch. We returned in time to conduct the last two days of the College. I wondered if people would recognize me when I returned, and expected that

I would have to reintroduce myself after being away from the group for more than three weeks. To my surprise, I was warmly greeted and welcomed back by both staff and students. They informed me that it had been a fantastic three weeks and excitedly proclaimed that it was all due to psychodrama. I could imagine that it had been an exciting and wonderful time; Spence had recruited some of the best known and most successful lawyers in the country as teachers. I was puzzled, however, that the success of the College was all attributed to psychodrama. I know how powerful psychodrama is but it seemed like three days out of 27 was hardly enough to have such a great impact. It took me some time to realize what had happened. Trial lawyers belong to an adversarial profession and lawyers tend to be competitive. They bring that attitude to an experience such as the College, hoping to stand out among their peers, wondering who their competition will be. During psychodrama they reveal and share their vulnerabilities as human beings, struggling with common problems of existence, striving to find their places in the world. Psychodrama reduces the competitiveness. Now, as several students have told me, "You didn't have to be better than anyone else. You only have to better than yourself when you came." John Ackerman, who served as an instructor at the College for many years, described the effect of psychodrama this way: "Psychodrama gets people opened up and teaches them how to be human beings, and then when we put them in these trial practice exercises they go at it in a human, caring, meaningful way" (Ackerman, 1998).

I returned to the 1995 session of the Trial Lawyers College prepared to stay and see how role training might be introduced. I observed how training was conducted and sometimes took part in the training activities. I discovered that six trial skills were taught: case analysis; voir dir; opening statement; direct examination, cross examination; and closing statement. The teaching method was a procedure that had been developed by another trial lawyer post-graduate training organization. Skill training was conducted in small groups of eight students, each with one or two instructors. Each student was asked to perform the skill being taught, e.g., "Give us ten minutes of an opening statement." After the student performed, the instructors and class members offered a critique, using the formula: "This is what I liked …", followed by "This is what (or how) I think you need to improve …"

This approach was certainly an advance over lectures but I thought that a role training design would be even more effective. In role training, the instructor/director can assist the student to improve *during* the action rather than giving suggestions *after* the action. The fact that students were active in the perform-and-critique procedure might make it relatively easy to shift to the role training method. The question in my mind was how to introduce a new way of teaching.

The answer came when Spence decided to bring back as instructors individuals who had attended the College as students. Sixteen people who had been students in the 1994 and 1995 programs were selected. I conducted a three day training workshop to introduce them to role training. They then attended the

1996 College as junior or assistant instructors, applying psychodrama techniques when they saw an opportunity.

In addition to what was happening at the Trial Lawyers College itself, psychodrama was having an effect beyond the College. Working reunions, initiated after the first session of Trial Lawyers College and later labeled Graduate Seminars, provided ongoing experience in psychodrama. Lawyers who were introduced to psychodrama through the college began attending the psychodrama training workshops of the National Psychodrama Training Center and eventually other training workshops for personal reasons.

A lawyer who had attended the 1994 class asked me to conduct psychodrama with several clients. He believed that they would achieve some emotional relief from the experiences that had made them his clients. I agreed to do so and worked with a number of his clients. They included four families with negligent death cases, each of whom had lost a member because someone's carelessness or neglect. The result, as the lawyer had hoped, was beneficial for the clients. There was also an unanticipated bonus. The psychodramas yielded valuable information about the case, heretofore unknown to the lawyer. A way to use psychodrama in trial preparation came to light.

The use of psychodrama at the Trial Lawyers College continued to grow. Each year more former students were invited to become instructors and attended a staff training week. More of the training was conducted psychodramatically. All case material used in demonstrations and in classroom work came from actual cases with which the student lawyers were working. Up to this time, the material had been presented as a fact pattern, a common term in law to describe the recitation of the salient features of a case. Two instructors of one small group were working with a student who was having a difficult time making a convincing opening statement. The instructors asked him to reverse roles with his client and reenact the major event upon which the lawsuit was based. The results were a marked improvement in the student's performance. After that, case material was presented by asking students to reverse roles with their clients, and reenact the essential events of the case. More ways of employing psychodrama techniques in preparation for trial were devised.

The indisputable advantage of reenactment over verbal description of a client's experience raised a question. Can lawyers use psychodrama with clients in discovering what had happened to them? In other words, can lawyers direct clients in psychodramatic reenactment? This issue is what makes the definition of psychodrama critical. If psychodrama is defined as a method of psychotherapy then it is unethical and illegal for someone not licensed to conduct psychotherapy to practice it. However, the American Board of Examiners in Psychodrama, Sociometry and Group Psychotherapy has a provision for certifying psychodramatists who are not psychotherapists. Additionally, I reasoned that if a professional person could ethically ask a client to *describe* to him or her what happened, that individual could ethically ask the client to *show* him or her what happened. However, there is a special caution for lawyers who conduct reenactments. One of the few dangers encountered in psychodramatic work is retraumatization by incompetent or careless reenactment of intense traumatic events. The situations which give rise to lawsuits are often decidedly traumatic. The lawyers of Trial Lawyers College are strongly advised to carefully consider the potential for retraumatizing a client and consult an experienced psychodramatist if there is a question. They are also encouraged to attend psychodrama training workshops to become proficient in directing if they wish to use psychodrama in trial preparation. Psychodrama became and remains an integral component of the Trial Lawyers College.

A common component of the trial lawyer's and the psychodrama director's task is story telling. Both take on the responsibility of telling the story of something that happened in the life of their respective clients. The legal profession has increasingly become aware of the importance of telling the client's story to the jury in a trial. Cole (2001) writes that

> There seems to be little dispute among trial lawyers and trial advocacy teachers that the essence of the trial is storytelling and that storytelling principles are not only helpful, but also essential to an engaging and persuasive presentation. Trial lawyers and trial advocacy teachers are looking for ways to take advantage of storytelling techniques to make our presentations more persuasive.
>
> *(p. 2)*

He backs up his assertion with a number of references. Gerry Spence was an early advocate and convinced practitioner of the storytelling strategy for conducting a trial. "You tell the story in voir dir," he told students. "You tell the story in your opening statement. You tell the story in examination of witnesses and in cross-examination. By the time of closing statements, you should have the story told." With respect to psychodrama, a classical psychodrama is typically the story of an event in the life of the protagonist. The director provides the tools for the protagonist to tell it in dramatic form. Those who have taken part in psychodrama know how compelling one's story is when acted out in a well-directed psychodrama. Lawyers long to be as convincing in the courtroom.

A trial lawyer has the responsibility for a client's well-being if he or she is trying a civil suit, or perhaps a client's freedom if it is a criminal trial. Persuasively telling the client's story improves the probability of repairing the harm done to the plaintiff. It increases the chances that an innocent person will not be punished unfairly. A compelling account of extenuating circumstances can help achieve an appropriate sentence for a guilty one. It is not surprising that trial lawyers are drawn to psychodrama, "the science which explores the truth by dramatic methods" (J. L. Moreno, 1946a, p. 249) or that they find psychodrama particularly appropriate for the practice of trial law.

The first aspect of psychodrama that attracts the lawyer to learn how to use psychodrama is the potential it has for trial preparation. However, the lawyers who then continue training in psychodrama inevitably report that the most important value they receive is personal growth. A frequent statement from many lawyers is "Psychodrama has changed everything that I do from the way I talk with a prospective client for the first time to the way I treat my paralegals and secretary to the way I treat my wife and children."

Interview with John Ackerman

In 1998, during the fifth year of the Trial Lawyers College, Dana Cole, who had been a student in 1995 and then made a staff instructor, conducted an interview with John Ackerman, who, as noted above, had introduced psychodrama into the legal profession. Cole graciously shared a transcript of that interview with me. Ackerman's thoughts are notable not only because of the history but with respect to his projections into the future.

Ackerman told Cole that when he became Dean of the National College of Criminal Defense in 1975, N.C.C.D. was a lecture program. He soon adopted the perform-and-critique method which is described above, in which students perform and then receive a critique of their performance. Although this approach was far superior to lecturing, Ackerman was not satisfied.

> I wanted to figure out a way to teach lawyers to be intuitive and creative and, and to just kind of understand at a, at a gut level that there were certain ways that would be effective in dealing with the trial of cases and dealing with juries.
>
> *(Ackerman, 1998, p. 9)*

He would not have known to phrase it this way but he wanted to teach lawyers to be spontaneous and creative.

Ackerman had a friend, John Johnson, a mental health worker from Wyoming where Ackerman grew up. Johnson and Ackerman had worked on a regionally famous case with Gerry Spence when Ackerman was a law student. He told Johnson what he wanted to do and asked if Johnson had any ideas. After some research, Johnson thought that psychodrama might be the answer, although he had no experience with the method. At an N.C.C.D. event, Ackerman, Johnson, and Spence, with Blatner's book, *Acting In* (1973), experimented with psychodrama. They concluded that it appeared to have promise but that a trained psychodramatist seemed advisable.

The first psychodrama workshop offered by the National College of Criminal Defense, advertised as "The Criminal Trial: A Psychodramatic Analysis" was held in Jackson, WY, in the fall of 1978. Don Clarkson was one of two psychodramatists engaged to direct it. Ackerman, Spence and Johnson presented the workshop with concern, Ackerman reports in the interview:

> We were pretty tentative about it. We didn't have a whole lot of confidence in it working. And for the first time I saw the immense power of psychodrama, just scared the crap out of me. Because by, oh, by mid afternoon on Friday, we had people getting involved in very intense personal psychodramas with all of the things that go along with that, and that was pretty scary. Because when you don't know much about psychodrama it, it almost looks dangerous.
>
> But we got through that two and a half days and the feedback we got from the people that had come was that it was just an absolutely fantastic experience. And in addition to dealing with personal psychodramas, we dealt a lot with problems people were having with cases they were involved in, problems with judges, problems with clients, things like that. And we were able to work through some things there that, that worked out quite well.
>
> *(Ackerman, 1998, pp. 16–17)*

Bolstered by the reception of the workshop, National College of Criminal Defense presented a number of similar workshops throughout the country. However, psychodrama did not become a part of the three-week summer program that the organization presented, Ackerman said "We maintained the normal summer program pretty much intact and saw psychodrama as some kind of a separate training thing and never worked the psychodramatic process into the summer training program, never did that" (p 17).

After Cole and Ackerman discuss the original use of psychodrama at the National College of Criminal Defense, and Ackerman's relationship with Gerry Spence and Trial Lawyers College where Ackerman was on the teaching staff, Cole asks Ackerman how the use of psychodrama has evolved. Ackerman replies that in the first year of the Trial Lawyers College, training began with three days of psychodrama. Then the lawyer training without psychodrama took place. There was still the separation between psychodrama and the teaching of trial skills:

> JOHN ACKERMAN: "It was psychodrama sits over here and teaches people and gets people opened up and teach[es] them how to be human beings, and then when we put them in these trial practice exercises they will go at it in a human, caring, meaningful way."
>
> DANA COLE: It worked, though; didn't it?
>
> JOHN ACKERMAN: Oh, the psychodrama was, was absolutely essential to, to what went on the rest of the time.
>
> *(p. 31)*

Cole asked how Ackerman sees the use of psychodrama evolving. Ackerman replied that until 1994, psychodrama was seen as an end in itself. The personal psychodrama experience makes for a better lawyer who:

> can stand up in front of a jury and be themselves and be honest (p. 33). It has evolved first into a way to train lawyers in trial skills, using the techniques of psychodrama throughout the training sessions. Then it has become a way for lawyers to take those techniques and prepare themselves for trial.
>
> And it's, it's ten times as powerful as we thought it was in the '70s in terms of what, what a marvelous tool it is for lawyers.
>
> I was remarking to John Nolte the other night that, having gone as far as we've gone with it, it makes me think that Moreno must have had lawyers in mind when he invented it, and that's not true, but I can't think of a profession where or a business or a calling where it can be such a useful and powerful and meaningful tool. I cannot think of one.
>
> *(pp. 33–34)*

Ackerman predicted that the use of psychodrama both in the training of trial lawyers and in trial preparation will continue to grow. He thought that the applications of psychodrama developed at the Trial Lawyers College will be adopted by law schools and other postgraduate lawyer training organizations. He foresees psychodrama training programs all over the country in the future. "This school [Trial Lawyers College] has taken the fear out of it. It's no longer a dirty word, I don't think, in lots of circles" (p. 37).

Finally, Ackerman in the interview says:

> I think it's just going to, we are going to keep developing and keep refining it. And one thing I'm reasonably certain about is we are going to, we are going to create a, a field of psychodrama that is a, a separate subspecialty of psychodrama that really involves lawyering and lawyer training and that over the next several years we are going to develop some, some enormously skillful trainers in that field.
>
> *(p. 47)*

The original Trial Lawyers College was conducted in 1994. Don Clarkson and I were the two psychodramatists. As psychodrama became integrated into the training program, Spence engaged additional psychodramatists, Kätlin Larimer in 1997 and Kathie St. Clare in 1999. Each of us made significant contributions to the Trial Lawyers College. All four of us have now retired from the College and other psychodramatists have taken our places. Trial Lawyers College conducts as many as 18 events a year, Regional Seminars, the 24-day College, Graduate Seminars, and others. Psychodrama is part of each one of them. Scores of lawyers who have attended TLC events have participated in additional psychodrama training programs. There are at least eight lawyers who are certified by the American Board of Examiners in Psychodrama, Sociometry and Group Psychotherapy, several of whom are certified at the advanced level of Trainer, Educator, and Practitioner. An estimated three to four thousand lawyers have experienced psychodrama through the Trial Lawyers Colleges many events. Psychodrama has become and remains an integral component of the Trial Lawyers College.

References

Ackerman, J. (1998). *Interview of John Ackerman at the Trial Lawyers College*. Dubois, Wyoming: Thunderhead Ranch. Unpublished interview.

Anna, B. (2003). Literature review of the integration of psychodramatic principles and practices in education. *Australian & New Zealand Psychodrama Association Journal*, 12, 62–84.

Blatner, A. (1973). *Acting-In: Practical Application of Psychodramatic Methods*. New York: Springer.

Campbell, A. (2012). Playing scientist: Using digital resources and role play to enhance student understanding of science as a human endeavor. *Science Scope*, 36(2), 31–35. Retrieved from www.jstor.org/stable/43184211.

Cole, D. (2001). Psychodrama and the training of trial lawyers: Finding the story. *Northern Illinois Law Review*, 21, 1–35.

Franz, J. G. (1939). Spontaneity training in public speaking classes: a preliminary report. *Sociometry*, 2, 49–53.

French, J. R. P. (1945). Role-playing as a method of training foremen. *Sociometry*, 8, 172–187.

Gartmeier, M., Bauer, J., Fischer, M., Hoppe-Seyler, T., Karsten, G., Kiessling, C. … Prenzel, M. (2015). Fostering professional communication skills of future physicians and teachers: effects of e-learning with video cases and role-play. *Instructional Science*, 43(4), 443–462. Retrieved from www.jstor.org/stable/43575299.

Haas, R. (1949a). Editor's foreword. In R. B. Haas (Ed.), *Psychodrama and Sociodrama in American Education*. Beacon, NY: Beacon House. VIII–XII.

Haas, R. B. (Ed.) (1949b). *Psychodrama and Sociodrama in American Education*. Beacon, NY: Beacon House.

Jacobs, J. (1945). The application of sociometry to industry. *Sociometry*, 8(2), 181–198.

Kassardjian, A., Rudrud, E., Taubman, M., Leaf, J., Edwards, A., Schulze, K. … Leaf, R. (2013). Utilizing teaching interactions to facilitate social skills in the natural environment. *Education and Training in Autism and Developmental Disabilities*, 48(2), 245–257. Retrieved from www.jstor.org/stable/23880643.

Kay, L. (1946). Role-playing as a teaching aid. *Sociometry*, 9(2/3), 263–274.

Kay, L. & Schick, J. (1945). Role-practice in training depth interviewers. *Sociometry*, 8, 82–85.

Lin, M., Lake, V. & Rice, D. (2008). Teaching anti-bias curriculum in teacher education programs: what and how. *Teacher Education Quarterly*, 35(2), 187–200. Retrieved from www.jstor.org/stable/23479231.

Lippitt, R. (1943). The psychodrama in leadership training. *Sociometry*, 6, 286–292.

Maier, N. (1952). *Principles of Human Relations: Applications to Management*. New York: John Wiley & Sons.

Maier, N. (1953). Dramatized case material as a springboard for role playing. *Group Psychotherapy*, 6, 30–42.

Maier, N. (1955a). *A Psychological Approach to Industrial Problems*. Boston, MA: Houghton Mifflin.

Maier, N. (1955b). *Psychology in Industry: A Psychological Approach to Industrial Problems* (2nd ed.). Boston, MA: Houghton Mifflin.

Maier, N. (1962). *Creative Management*. New York: John Wiley & Sons.

Maier, N. (1965). *Psychology in Industry*. Boston, MA: George G. Harrap & Co.

Maier, N. (1975). *Role Play Technique: Handbook for Management and Leadership Practice*. La Jolla, CA: University Associates.

Maier, N., Solem, A. & Maier, A. (1957). *Supervisory and Executive Development: A Manual for Role Playing*. New York: Wiley.

Miller, D. C. (1951). Introductory demonstrations and applications of three major uses of role playing for business and government administrators. *Sociometry*, 14, 48–58.

Moreno, J. L. (1934). *Who Shall Survive? A New Approach to the Problems of Human Interrelations*. Washington, DC: Nervous and Mental Disease Publishing Company.

Moreno, J. L. (1946a). Psychodrama and group psychotherapy. *Sociometry*, 9, 249–253.

Moreno, J. L. (1946b). *Psychodrama, First Volume*. Beacon, NY: Beacon House.

Moreno, J. L. (1947a). Foundations of sociatry. *Sociatry*, 1, 10–15.

Moreno, J. L. (1947b). *The Theatre of Spontaneity*. Beacon, NY: Beacon House.

Moreno, J. L. (1953a). Preludes of the sociometric movement. In J. L. Moreno, *Who Shall Survive?* (pp. 13–108). Beacon, NY: Beacon House.

Moreno, J. L. (1953b). *Who Shall Survive?* Beacon, NY: Beacon House.

Moreno, J. L. (1989). The autobiography of J. L. Moreno, MD (Abridged). *Group Psychotherapy, Psychodrama & Sociometry*, 42, 3–52.

Moreno, J. L. & Jennings, H. (1936). Spontaneity training, a method of personality development. *Sociometric Review*, 17–25.

Moreno, Z. T. (1967). The seminal mind of J. L. Moreno and his influence upon the present generation. *International Journal of Sociometry and Sociatry*, 5, 145–156.

Rogers, M. (1946). Problems of human relations in industry. *Sociometry*, 9(4), 350–371.

Shaftel, F. & Shaftel, G. (1982). *Role Playing in the Curriculum* (2nd ed.). Englewood Cliffs, NJ: Prentice-Hall.

Shearon, E. M. & Shearon, W. (1973). Some uses of psychodrama in education. *Group Psychotherapy & Psychodrama*, 26, 47–52.

Shoobs, N. (1943). The psychodramatic approach to classroom problems. *Sociometry*, 6(3), 264–265.

Shoobs, N. (1944). Psychodrama in the schools. *Sociometry*, 7(2), 152–168.

Shoobs, N. (1947). Sociometry in the class room. *Sociometry*, 10, 154–164.

Simpson, J. & Elias, V. (2011). Choices and chances: the sociology role-playing game—The sociological imagination in practice. *Teaching Sociology*, 39(1), 42–56. Retrieved from www.jstor.org/stable/41308923.

Sternberg, P. & Garcia, A. (1989). *Sociodrama: Who's in Your Shoes?* Westport, CT: Praeger.

Yunker, M., Orion, N. & Lernau, H. (2011). Merging playfulness with the formal science curriculum in an outdoor learning environment. *Children, Youth and Environments*, 21 (2), 271–293. Retrieved from www.jstor.org/stable/10.7721/chilyoutenvi.21.2.0271.

Zander, A. F. & Lippitt, R. (1944). Reality-practice as method. *Sociometry*, 7, 129–151.

7

PSYCHODRAMA THEORY

I agree with Kellermann (1992) when he writes that psychodramatists appear to have a much greater interest in the practice of the method than in theory and research. However I take issue with his statement that psychodrama theory is "a hodgepodge of unrelated thoughts, unintegrated by any one systematic framework" (p. 33). I suspect that impression comes from the challenge of understanding J. L. Moreno's writing and the fact that Moreno's contributions are founded in existential, phenomenological philosophy rather than the positivist, objectivist, reductionist philosophy upon which the natural sciences are based.

Philosophical Basis of Psychodrama

Psychodrama has its origin in existential philosophy and is an existential, phenomenological method. This differentiates psychodramatic psychotherapy from most conventional methods, even those identified as existential therapies, and from the medical model of mental illness, both of which are grounded in a positivist, reductionist philosophy. This distinction also helps explain why psychodrama has never been more than a marginal component of the mental health professions despite the fact that many of Moreno's innovations have been widely adopted by non-psychodramatic therapists. It is also why psychodramatic theory is often poorly understood even by practicing psychodramatists.

J. L. Moreno, as were many of his European peers in the early years of the twentieth century, was profoundly influenced by the existential philosophy of Søren Kirkegaard. Moreno distinguished between Kirkegaardian existentialism, the intellectual existentialism of philosophers, and "heroic" existentialism. He described the former as Kirkegaard's protest against the hypocritical religion of Kirkegaard's time. Intellectual existentialism is the philosophical discussion and analysis of existential themes such as being, death, meaning, etc. Moreno (1956) described heroic existentialism as living out Being as Kirkegaard dreamed of doing rather than discussing it as philosophers do. The aim of Moreno and his four companions of the Religion of Encounter was to live fully in the moment. Moreno described them as making, "One of the most concentrated attempts at a heroic life … which combined a high degree of awareness with action, integrating existence with knowledge …" (p. 61). Their first basic principle was the all- inclusiveness of being and the constant effort to maintain from moment to moment the natural, spontaneous, uninterrupted flow of existence. The second principle was the notion that all existing things were good in and of themselves. Other concepts included the notion of the moment, the idea of the situation, and the conviction that conduct should be based on Spontaneity-Creativity rather than on ethical and cultural conserves. "And above all, the urgency, the urgency of their immediate experience" (J. L. Moreno, 1989, p. 48). All of Moreno's later methods and theory were based, he says, upon these ideas.

From the theoretical Canon of Spontaneity, intrinsic in all Morenean contributions, to the physical creation of dramas from the subjective experience of a protagonist, psychodrama is existential and phenomenological. This fact has caused confusion for those trained in other modalities who attempt to understand psychodrama from a traditional scientific orientation based on the positivistic, deterministic, objective, reductionist philosophical approach. Although conventional science has been enormously productive in the physical and biological sciences, questions have long been raised about its appropriateness in social and psychological science.

The differences between the two philosophical positions begins with the basic way in which each looks at the issue of understanding human behavior. Traditional psychology regards the individual as *an organism in an environment.* From the perspective of the radical behaviorism of B. F. Skinner, human behavior is absolutely determined and under control of the environment through the contingencies of reinforcement. This school of behaviorism that is quite influential in the field of psychology considers mental activities such as thinking, planning, remembering, or dreaming as epiphenomena, secondary effects that have no causal influence themselves. Psychology, once considered the science of the mind, is now defined as the science of behavior. The major method of studying behavior is through making changes in some aspect of the environment and measuring the response of subject.

Opposed to this position is the existential, phenomenological position of psychodrama that considers the individual as *a being in a situation.* The individual is a thinking, feeling, remembering, acting, holistic being who brings the consequences of life experiences into the situation. Moreno was not interested is responses to stimuli but in acts, complex and purposeful behavior intended to achieve a specific result. The *situation* involves not only the physical environment in which we happen to be in the moment, but also how we happen to be where we are. Each situation includes a challenge, a demand for action, a need or desire to achieve. The situation also comprises the other people with whom to interact to meet the challenge or to fulfill the need or desire. The conventional psychological model is a deterministic, mechanical model of human behavior. The existential psychodramatic one is a non-deterministic (spontaneous), dynamic one.

Canon of Spontaneity–Creativity

Creativity has forever been a preoccupation of humankind. Every society has a story to account for the creation of the world and of humankind. "Creativity is the problem of the universe; it is, therefore, the problem of all existence, the problem of every religion, science, the problem of psychology, sociometry and human relations," J. L. Moreno wrote (1955b, p. 382). It was during Moreno's engagement with children in the *Augarten* of Vienna, about 1911, that the concept of spontaneity began to form and the seeds of his theory of spontaneity–creativity were sown. The conventional strategy for creativity research has focused on the individuals who have made outstanding contributions in their respective fields of endeavor, people whom we consider to exemplify creative behavior. Artists of all media, authors, painters, and sculptors are examples. The philosophers who publish new ideas and scientists who make new discoveries or publish grand new theories are considered paragons of creativity. Creativity in this sense is regarded as a talent or personality trait or some special gift that sets these individuals apart from others. Moreno had a different idea. He sought to devise and articulate a common process to explain how everything, from stars and planets to the evolution of new species, to the emergence of new theories, to the everyday creativity of ordinary human beings, came into existence. Although he had perceived the association of spontaneity with creativity early, perhaps by 1911 or 1912, Moreno first published the Canon of Creativity in *Who Shall Survive?* (1953, p. 46). It is reproduced in Figure 7.1.

There are four concepts basic to the Canon of Creativity: the conserve, creativity, spontaneity, and the warming up process. According to the Canon, a creative act begins with warming up signaling the presence of spontaneity. Spontaneity, a novel and appropriate response to the situation, interacts with creativity and produces a conserve. As presented by Moreno, The Canon of Creativity is sparse and compact. Moreno complicates matters by scattering his discussions of spontaneity, creativity, the conserve, and the warming up process throughout a number of different articles and books. The following discussion represents my understanding of Moreno's Canon of Spontaneity–Creativity.

CANON OF CREATIVITY

SPONTANEITY - CREATIVITY - CONSERVE

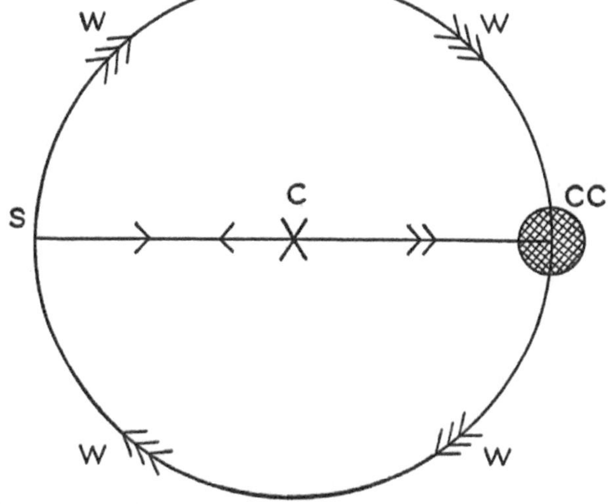

FIELD OF ROTATING OPERATIONS BETWEEN SPONTANEITY-CREATIVITY-CULTURAL CONSERVE (S-C-CC)

S—Spontaneity, C—Creativity, CC—Cultural (or any) Conserve (for instance, a biological conserve, *i.e.*, an animal organism, or a cultural conserve, *i.e.*, a book, a motion picture, or a robot, *i.e.*, a calculating machine); W—Warming up is the "operational" expression of spontaneity. The circle represents the field of operations between S, C and CC.

Operation I: Spontaneity arouses Creativity, C. S——> C.

Operation II: Creativity is receptive to Spontaneity. S <——C.

Operation III: From their interaction Cultural Conserves, CC, result. S——> C——>> CC.

Operation IV: Conserves (CC) would accumulate indefinitely and remain "in cold storage". They need to be reborn, the catalyzer Spontaneity revitalizes them. CC——>>> S——>>> CC.

S does not operate in a vacuum, it moves either towards Creativity or towards Conserves.

Total Operation

Spontaneity-creativity-warming up act< actor / conserve

From Moreno, J. L. "Who Shall Survive?", 2nd Edition, 1953, page 46.

FIGURE 7.1 Canon of Creativity

The Conserve

A conserve is defined by Moreno as the end result of a creative act. Anything that has been created is a conserve. Thus every *thing* in the universe is a conserve. Every noun in the dictionary identifies a conserve. a special category of the conserve is the *cultural conserve* which refers to humanly created conserves. The various forms of shelter, societies, tools and instruments, technologies, as well as all works of art, disciplines of study, religions, and theories of all kinds are cultural conserves. Of special interest to the psychodramatist are roles, role relationships, and interpersonal interactions. These, too, are cultural conserves.

Creativity

Synonyms for creativity in everyday language are inventiveness, imagination, innovation, and originality, traits or characteristics of individuals who are seen as creative. Moreno has an entirely different concept of creativity. "Creativity," he writes, "belongs to the categories of substance—it is the arch substance ..." (J. L. Moreno, 1953, p. 40.) "The universe is infinite creativity" and "Creativity is the ever nourishing maternal center." "In order to become effective it (the sleeping beauty) needs a catalyzer" (J. L. Moreno, 1955a, p. 359). That catalyzer, of course, is spontaneity. These thoughts convey a sense of creativity but to me, they are indeterminate and nebulous descriptions. I have come to the conclusion that creativity in the Morenean sense can best be understood as the *potential for becoming*, the possibility for being created. Understood this way, creativity at the moment just prior to the Big Bang included every thing that has since been created by nature or by man. This includes the universe and everything in the universe. It encompasses all the features of the physical and the biological worlds. It includes all human creations as sketched out above: tools and implements, technologies, scientific discoveries and theories, all the works of art, paintings, sculptures, books, poems, religions and philosophies, all languages, alphabets and words, all symbols and concepts, and roles that now exist or have ever existed. These entities were once potentially possible. Once manifested, they become conserves.

Creativity of course is not limited to that which has been created. Moreno pointed out that the Biblical account of creation of the universe in six days can't be accurate. The universe is still being created and, as far as can be imagined, will continue to be under construction infinitely. Creativity, therefore, encompasses all those conserves that will eventually be created, both by nature and by man. If the universe is non-determinate, as both Moreno (1946) and quantum mechanics maintain, there is another category of creativity. There must be conserves of all kinds that could have been created but were not, species of animals and plants, scientific theories, mathematical formulas, books, languages and so forth that were potentially capable of coming into being in the past but which did not, or capable of coming into being in the future but which will not. They, none the less, belong to the category of creativity.

Spontaneity

It is in the presence of spontaneity that conserves emerge from the potential of creativity into reality. Spontaneity is the catalyzer required for the conserve to emerge from the maternal center of creativity, to awaken the sleeping beauty, in Moreno's words. Moreno variably characterized spontaneity as a catalyst, as energy, and as a response. Spontaneity is like a catalyst in that it enters into and influences the creative process without itself undergoing a permanent change. There is a problem with considering spontaneity as a response which I will explain below. The most appropriate way to describe spontaneity seems to be as a kind of energy.

Spontaneity is, however, a very special form of energy according to Moreno. Spontaneity is *unconservable energy*. That statement is an oxymoron from the purview of classical physics. The law of conservation of energy holds that energy can be neither created or destroyed. Energy can only be transformed from one kind to another, from electrical energy to light energy, for example. Moreno agreed that physical and mental energy *is* conservable, but that it is the unconservable spontaneity that is responsible for the creativity in the universe.

Spontaneity–creativity theory requires rejection of the doctrine of absolute determinism and Moreno adopted a rule of partial determinism for the world in which we live (J. L. Moreno, 1946, pp. 102–103, 1953, pp. 43–35). Moreno gave credit to French philosopher Henri Bergson (Bergson & Mitchell, 1911/1944) for introducing the notion of spontaneity into philosophy: "To Henri Bergson, for one, goes the honor of having brought the principle of spontaneity into philosophy (although he rarely used the word), at a time when the leading scientists were adamant that there is no such thing in objective science" (J. L. Moreno, 1946, p. 8). Like Moreno, Bergson rejected the principle of absolute determinism.

Students and colleagues initially had difficulty in grasping Moreno's notion of spontaneity, especially from his metaphorical descriptions such as "Creativity is the ever nourishing maternal center; spontaneity the ever moving masculine fertilizer …" (1955a, p. 359). Moreno finally adopted a definition that he termed "operational" and which he phrased in several ways: "Spontaneity is the variable degree of adequate response to a situation of a variable degree of novelty" (1953, p. 722). Moreno gave this definition in several different versions, e.g.: "We have called this response of an individual to a new situation—and the new response to an old situation–spontaneity" (J. L. Moreno, 1946, p. 50); and "Spontaneity operates in the present, now and here; it propels the individual towards an adequate response to a new situation or new response to an old situation" (J. L. Moreno, 1953, p. 42). Kipper (1967) and I (Nolte, 2014) have both criticized this definition on the grounds that responses are observable while energy is not. Spontaneity, a form of energy, therefore cannot be an observable response. Kipper has suggested that confusion between spontaneity and the warming up process has resulted in attributes of the warming up process being attributed to spontaneity. A response, then, reflects the effect of spontaneity, not spontaneity itself, and belongs to the concept of the warming up process. Moreno's definition does, however, invoke the two attributes that characterize the presence of spontaneity in the response, novelty and adequacy.

Moreno recognized that his concept of spontaneity did not fall within the realm of possibility as far as classical physics was concerned (J. L. Moreno, 1955e). This fact did not shake his confidence in the reality of it. He suggested that quantum theory might one day be able to explain spontaneity. In another work, I have suggested that this has already occurred. It is my opinion that David Bohm's concept of the quantum potential, an energy significantly different from the various forms of energy of classical physics, is the energy that Moreno labeled spontaneity. I believe that Bohm's (1980) theory of the implicate order offers a quantum theory version of Moreno's Canon of Creativity (Nolte, 2014, Chapter 6).

From Moreno's perspective, spontaneity is not just responsible for human creativity. It functions throughout the universe, in the creation of stars and planets, and in nature. Spontaneity is involved in the change in geometrical features of the earth. Spontaneity results in the evolution of animals and plants. Spontaneity plays a role in the genesis of every individual of every species of plant and animal.

Warming Up Process

The warming up phase of a psychodrama session has been discussed in Chapter 3 of this book. The more theoretical *warming up process* is considered here. The warming up process is defined by Moreno (1953) as "the *operational* expression of spontaneity. Spontaneity and warming up process operate on all levels of human relations, eating, walking, sleeping, sexual intercourse, social communication, creativity, in religious self realization and asceticism." (p. 42). In at least one passage, Moreno (1955d) suggested that spontaneity was observable. Conceived of as a form of energy, spontaneity itself is invisible. Like all forms of energy, spontaneity is identified by its effects. The warming up process, then, is the observable effects of the presence to spontaneity, just like light or heat are the observable effects of electricity.

"The warming up process manifests itself in every expression of the living organism *as it strives towards an act.* It has a somatic expression, a psychological expression, and a social expression" (J. L. Moreno & F. B. Moreno, 1944, p. 98). "We are never in action without some warming up to it" (J. L. Moreno, 1946, p. 56). The warming up process is a general condition existing before and in the course of any creative act—before and during an act of sleeping, eating, sexual intercourse, walking, artistic creation, or any act of self realization. Warming up precedes the act and continues throughout the action.

Warming up can be thought of as preparation to act. Both individuals and groups warm up to action. Moreno (1955d) identified five types of warming up. The first is *undirected warming up*, typified by "vague, chaotic, confused, moving towards several goals on several tracks simultaneously" (p. 368). One can observe both groups and individuals warming up in this manner.

An individual or group in a *directed warming up process* appears to be proceeding smoothly and clearly toward an action. Preceding the directed warming up, there may be a period of organizing perceptual cues as one seeks to:

> find the melody which fits into his musical composition or to find a mathematical formula for a hypothetical question or to find an ending for

> a poem or an answer to his wife's quarrels. As soon as he is sure what to do, he has sudden flashes of perception, then he acts quickly-registers the ending of the poem in his mind, rushes to the piano and tries the melody, writes a letter resigning from his job or talks to his wife, etc.
>
> *(p. 368)*

Moreno also recognized a condition that he called *a general state of warm up*. This is typical of individuals facing a new and unknown situation. The first day in a new job or going on a blind date are examples of such situations. Anticipation is the common emotion.

Emergency situations can result in *immediate warming up*. The driver of a car about to be in an accident may take evasive action and escape the crash. The driver reports that he acted without thinking about it. This reflects immediate warming up. This kind of warming up is also common in heroic actions.

The last type of warming up process that Moreno described was the *chain warm up*. Here an idea or a feeling is initiated by one individual and suggested to another who passes it along to a third. It travels from one member of a group to the next, building up intensity until it comes back to the initiator. This, wrote Moreno, is a common process in group decision making. Suggestions are expressed until one of them attracts adherents and is repeated and amplified. The group is then warmed up and goes into action.

Moreno (1955b) illustrated his personal warming up process in an article which was a reply to a paper submitted for publication in *Sociometry* by his friend and colleague, Pitirim Sorokin. Sorokin, a friendly colleague, Harvard professor, and like Moreno, a student of creativity had submitted a paper (Sorokin, 1955) in which he criticized Moreno's linking of spontaneity and creativity. Moreno pondered how he could illustrate that linkage. He decided that the way was to describe his warming up process to the writing of his reply to Sorokin in that reply.

He begins with the question: "How did the writing of this article come about?" It began with the receipt and reading of Sorokin's paper Moreno noted. It is not Sorokin himself, but a product of Sorokin's creativity, a cultural conserve, that starts things off. In his Canon of Creativity, Moreno points out that cultural conserves, an address or piece of writing, can serve to initiate the warming up process to action on the part of others. A patriotic poster, for example, can lead people to enlisting in the army. Receiving Sorokin's paper in the mail warmed Moreno up to the act of reading it. As Moreno reads Sorokin's paper, he writes, he "lifts" it from the paper upon which it is written and reproduces it in his mind. Because at this point it is a conserve, Sorokin cannot add anything to the article, no matter how many times Moreno reads it. Repeated reading may make it become clearer in Moreno's mind but will not extend or change it.[1]

As he reads the paper, Moreno begins to react to the article. All kinds of ideas come to him. He thinks, "Sorokin is right about that" on a certain point; and "Sorokin clearly misunderstands the concept of spontaneity, but this is not too serious." Moreno is well warmed up to reading the article. It has claimed his full attention. Then:

> But suddenly I read a sentence about *creative* "conserves" which alarms me. Conserves by themselves without an "intervening" factor do not become creative. We build up the conserves and try to make them look like idols. I see the ghosts of Plato and Aristotle coming back. It makes creativity look stale and it makes a puppet out of God. No! No! Aristotle and Plato have idolized the conserve like hundreds of other philosophers of Western civilization, including Spinoza, for whom God became a huge existential conserve, similar to St. John's logos [for] whom "The Word" implies an eternal, unchangeable conserve; here he was betraying Jesus who was intuitively set against it. More than the creators, we admire their conserves until they become sacred, like the "Bible", Beethoven's music or the "Pyramids".
>
> *(1955b, p. 383)*

Now Moreno's warm up changes. He makes an immediate decision that he *must* answer Sorokin. Until now his warming up has been only to the act of reading Sorokin's paper. Perceiving the phrase, "creative conserves," shifts his warm up to another action. His warm up now becomes directed towards another goal, writing a reply to Sorokin.

A number of new thoughts run through his mind as the obstacles to writing an article at this time occur to him: His secretary is sick and may not be able to work for some days. There is a deadline for submission of articles to the journal. He has a lecture which gives him little time. He feels tired and overburdened. His wife wants them to take a vacation. These thoughts are "*part* of my warming up process which is the operational manifestation of spontaneity. The sum of it is that I am gradually getting ready to write. I am only uncertain as to *what* I should say beyond what I have said so many times" (p. 384). Then inspiration strikes. Moreno decides to start his response to Sorokin's critique by describing his warming up process to the writing of that very response. In that way, perhaps, he can make the relationship between spontaneity, creativity and the conserve more comprehensible to Sorokin and other readers. It was that inspiration, to give an existential account of his warming up process to writing the response, that set him off to create it. "It is like suddenly finding the key to a musical composition or the essential line for a poem" (p. 384).

The Moment

Moreno's concept of the moment is a closely related to spontaneity. It is not a unit of time but the experience of the immediate, of the here and now. The moment is more than "a fleeting transition between past and future" (1946, p. 105). It is of a different quality than either the past or the present. In the existentialism of Moreno, the past is memory-in-the-moment of past experiences; the future is here and now anticipation-in-the-moment of what might be eventually experienced. The following three elements have to be present for the moment to be experienced: change, novelty, and activity.

A psychodrama is a spontaneously created drama, created in the moment. This is so even if scenes in the drama are re-enactments of events that the protagonist experienced earlier in life. We are not actually reenacting past experiences; rather we are enacting the protagonist's here-and-now memory of past experiences. The same holds true for future projections. We are enacting the protagonist's here-and-now anticipations of what the future may bring. We can only act in the moment, not in memory, not in imagination, not in anticipation.

The Situation

The situation includes the physical and social environment and the meaning that it has for the individual. The individual is not only a human being, but also a particular human being in this moment. One brings into the situation the residual effects of and the learning from all the situations which one has previously experienced and which have led the individual into the present situation. This includes attitudes and conclusions that one has drawn about oneself, about people in general, about the universe and how one is positioned in it. These all play a role in one's interpretation of the situation one is in. The individual's interpretation of the situation and the individual's goals, desires, and expectations influence the acts and actions of the individual. Human behavior, however, is not absolutely determined; it is *partially* determined and there is the possibility of original actions *not* determined by the past. Every individual has a unique history of experiences, every individual-in-a-situation is a unique event. The psychodrama itself is a unique event and it can only take place in the here-and-now.

Psychodrama can be studied by conventional research methods, of course, and Moreno encouraged such research. As a matter of fact, psychodrama provides a means for the study of subjective events, not otherwise susceptible to objective research methods, by transforming them into observable action. However, from a Morenean point of view the individual, social groups, behavior, psychopathology, and psychotherapy are perceived differently from the way they are regarded from a traditional scientific perspective. This fact has caused confusion for those who have been trained in other modalities before they come to psychodrama.

Action Theory

Action. J. L. Moreno had a brilliant inspiration when he decided to alleviate the marriage problems of a *Stegreiftheater* actress by premeditated assignment of roles that would allow her to act out the behaviors that were threatening her relationship with her husband. In doing so, he introduced action into the restoration of emotional equilibrium. He engaged the whole person in the psychotherapeutic process. Describing a life experience, as one does in verbal psychotherapy, is quite different from reenacting it. A verbal account is an abstraction of the experience. It is like the difference between watching a hurricane on TV and being in one. Protagonists re-living a past experience tend to dispense with evasions and equivocations that are easy to invoke, even unwittingly in the privacy of the psychotherapist's office. *Reenacting* a life event awakens the original emotions and feelings that are associated with it in ways that *talking about* it cannot. "However important verbal behavior is, *the act is prior to the word*, and 'includes' it" (J. L. Moreno, 1955c, p. 17).

The psychoanalysts attempt to understand the analysand's behavior, and especially unconscious motivations, from free associations and by interpreting dreams. Clinical psychologists attempt to understand and predict behavior by interpreting the responses that subjects make to various tests and inventories. Experimental psychologists devise prescribed tasks by which they can analyze behavior into its basic components. Moreno asked his subjects to act out their experiences, fantasies, and dreams. Psychodrama involves the actual behavior of subjects in life like situations. It is modeled after life itself.

J. L. Moreno (1955b) pointed out that watching an individual reenacting an experience, fantasy, or dream on the psychodrama stage provided far more information about that person than could be obtained from free association, interview, or tests. Verbal descriptions convey life in an intellectual sense, not as it is embodied in action. Describing one's experience, as is done in verbal psychotherapy, is quite different from acting it out; a verbal account is an abstraction of that experience. Making an experience concrete and tangible in psychodrama allows us to understand it in great depth. The flexibility of psychodrama permits a comprehensive and detailed exploration of life events. Psychodramatic action involves the whole person, cognition, memory, emotion, and the physical body, not simply recall. It requires no elaborate theory of the mind or hypotheses of how various experiences influence one's behavior and outlook on life. These phenomena are made manifest and evident. "Acting out within a therapeutic setting is the therapeutic counterpart of living itself. It cannot be substituted by any form of 'interpretation' even if the therapist were God himself" (J. L. Moreno, 1960a).

One of Sigmund Freud's major contributions to psychology was his discovery of the importance of unconscious motivation in understanding psychopathology and human behavior in general. Moreno applauded Freud's contribution while rejecting Freud's model of the unconscious as a locked container. Moreno hypothesized a continuum from *fully aware* to *unconscious of*, and held that we have varying degrees of awareness of the urges and desires that move us into action, a notion that is now widely held. The hidden dynamics of behavior are better brought to view in action than in words because acting is closer to the deeper levels of that which is unconscious than is language. The more involved the individual becomes in the action, the less aware he or she is of his or her actions. "It is like seeing the acting out of the unconscious itself" (p. 14). It is clear to Moreno that "the inclusion of the motor end of the psychic apparatus into the system of the [unconscious] becomes a foregone conclusion" (p. 17). The differences between verbal methods and psychodrama are so stark that psychodrama might better be considered as an alternative to psychotherapy rather than as a method of psychotherapy.

Psychodramatic action mitigates the issue of transference as it confronts conventional psychoanalysts and psychotherapists. By putting the individual into action on the psychodrama stage with auxiliaries in the roles of the significant figures in the protagonist's life, the protagonist is allowed, expected, and encouraged to express feelings of love and hate openly and overtly. These feelings are not transference; they are real feelings of love and hate. This way, transference onto the therapist is greatly reduced or eliminated.

For the conventional psychotherapist acting out is perceived as resistance to therapy. Acting out in this context refers to impulsive behaviors that a client engages in rather than dealing with the underlying motivations in the therapy session. Moreno maintained that acting out in the controlled setting of psychodrama not only provided more information but also served to reduce the potential for impulsive acting out in life situations.

Act Hunger

Everybody is expected to live up to his official role in life—a teacher is to act as a teacher, a pupil as a pupil, and so forth. But the individual craves to embody far more roles than those he is allowed to act out in life and even one or more varieties within the same role. Every individual is filled with different roles which he wants to become active in and that are present in him in different stages of development. It is from the active pressure which these multiple individual units exert upon the manifest official role that a feeling of anxiety is often produced (J. L. Moreno, 1953, p. 535).

Moreno called these cravings act hunger and according to him, act hunger exemplifies the infant, accounting for the fact that we have so little memory of events we have experienced before the age of about three. "The act-hunger of the infant is so great and so incessant that he uses all his energy up for this and as little as possible, for such an apparently negligible thing as remembering (this remembering is done by the auxiliary ego for him)" (J. L. Moreno, F. B. Moreno, 1944, p. 108). Young children are full of act hunger, as they strive to get the measure of this strange world into which they have been dropped and conquer it. They inevitably wish to accomplish tasks far beyond their abilities. We see the act hunger in four or five year old children pushing their toy lawnmowers behind their fathers' gas powered machines, and in their helping mothers stir cake batter or roll out pie dough (and licking the pans and spoons clean, of course.) The appeal of superheroes to children reflects the hunger for the strength and power that they can realize only in fantasy.

Act hunger does not disappear in adulthood.

> Every one of us has ideas—"dreams"—of himself in a variety of situations. These we call "roles". Most of our roles remain in the "dream" stage—they are never attempted or begun, and any attempts at actualizing our roles … remain, like most of our relationships, fragmentary, inconclusive, loose ends.
>
> *(J. L. Moreno, 1940a, p. 228)*

The fictional Walter Mitty (Thurber, 1939) is the embodiment of act hunger, and we all recognize ourselves to some degree in his story.

Recognition and acceptance of reality causes us to suppress many of our secret wishes, making our act hungers to be less visible than they are in childhood. However, most adults could, if they desired, acknowledge that they have had fantasies of greatness, of winning acclaim or accomplishing formidable feats, if not in football, baseball, tennis, or golf, then in an academic field, politics, in business or industry, or on the battlefield.

We are all Walter Mittys and we all experience the tensions of act hunger. The psychodrama stage offers a special world in which we can experience those roles that are otherwise forbidden us. For example, a mother may meet and embrace the children that she dreamed of but which her body could not produce. An accountant can become a cosmonaut. A man can give birth to a baby. One can travel the entire earth. The possibilities are infinite.

Surplus Reality

Children discovered it long before Moreno labeled it surplus reality. Cops and Robbers, Cowboys and Indians, House, School, War, Space Explorer, and dozens of other creative activities permit the players to have adventures, create roles, and visit places that are way beyond their abilities in the ordinary reality of life. The virtual reality of psychodrama allows adults, too, the freedom to experience over and above the reality of everyday living. The term, surplus reality, Moreno wrote, was inspired by Marx's concept of surplus value, that part of the earnings which the capitalist employer takes from the worker. Surplus reality, however, is not a loss but an enrichment of reality based on imagination.

Moreno described the surplus reality of the psychodrama stage thus:

> It provides the actor with a living space which is multi-dimensional and flexible to the maximum. The living space of reality is often narrow and restraining; he may easily lose his equilibrium. On the stage he may find

> it again, due to its methodology of freedom—freedom from unbearable stress and freedom for experience and expression. The stage space is an extension of life beyond the reality test of life itself. Reality and fantasy are not in conflict, but both are functions within a wider sphere—the psychodramatic world of objects, persons and events. The architectural design of the stage is made in accord with operational requirements. The stage's circular forms and levels—levels of aspiration—point up to the vertical dimension, stimulate relief from tensions and permit mobility and flexibility of action. High above the stage is the balcony level from where the megalomaniac, the Messiah, the hero, communicates with the group. The space surrounding the stage is designed to contain the group.
> *(J. L. Moreno, 1953, p. 82)*

Psychodrama provides a medium that is modeled after life but which provides for a more extensive reality than is possible in life. On the psychodrama stage the protagonist can re-visit experiences from the past, confront inter- or intra-personal conflicts in a controlled way, or explore anticipations of the future. The protagonist can return to any place he or she has ever been or wishes to be, the house one lived in as a child which is no longer standing, one's office, or a private island in the South Pacific. Indeed, the protagonist can conjure up any place on earth, on Mars, the moon, or in the cosmos, heaven or hell. One can encounter the parent who has been dead for many years, friends who have not been seen for too long a time, current relationships, and even one's hallucinations and delusions. All manner of experiences which everyday reality will not permit are possible of realization in surplus reality. "Hence, psychodrama brings the entire cosmos into play" (J. L. Moreno, 1965, p. 213).

Psychodramatists often reserve the term surplus reality for psychodramatic scenes that are not based on an event from the protagonist's life. This is not strictly accurate since all of psychodrama is actually surplus reality. In role reversal, the protagonist becomes someone else with whom he or she is related. Every psychodramatic technique invokes an element of surplus reality. Auxiliary egos and empty chairs represent individuals. Protagonists are permitted to encounter those people who are dead. Males can become females and vice versa. It is through surplus reality that the protagonist can achieve new, reorganized perceptions of self, significant others, relationships, and status in the world (Z. T. Moreno, Blomkvist, & Reutzel, 2000).

Role Theory

"The concept underlying this approach is the recognition that *man is a role player*, that every individual is characterized by a certain range of roles which dominate his behavior, and that every culture is characterized by a certain set of roles which it imposes with a varying degree of success upon its membership" (J. L. Moreno, 1961, p. 518). Role is the functioning form the individual assumes in the specific moment he reacts to a specific situation in which other persons or objects are involved.

"Role is a fusion of private and collective elements" (J. L. Moreno, 1960b, p. 80). There is the collective social role of, for instance, *the* mother, *the* doctor, *the* storekeeper. There are also the multitude of ways in which individuals create and take the roles of mother, doctor, and storekeeper. Roles relate individuals to each other and to their culture, to society.

All relationships can be described in terms of role and a role implies a complementary role. There is no parental role without a child role, an employer role without an employee role, or a doctor role without a patient role. In a role relationship, each person has expectations of how the other will act. In a successful transaction, both members achieve a goal and a change takes place in the situation.

Some roles are heavily prescribed by social custom and convention as well as by legal definition. The roles of physician, judge, teacher, and minister are some examples. No matter how rigid these prescriptions may be, considerable latitude is given to and expected from the individual acting in one of these roles. Every individual who takes the role of a doctor does so in a way which is different in some degree from every other doctor. However, if the individual behaves too differently from most other doctors, patients, will wonder if this really is a doctor, no matter what diplomas hang on the walls.

There is a reciprocal process in interpersonal interactions. The expectations that each member has of the other influences the other's behavior. There is also a reciprocal process between individuals and society. Social roles both guide and dictate how one takes or creates an individual role. At the same time, the way in which individuals create and take roles expands and revises, and sometimes transforms, the social role.

Moreno classified roles as psychosomatic, psychodramatic, and social roles. The psychosomatic roles are the first to emerge and are associated with physiological and physical functions. They include the role of the eater, the defecator, the sleeper, etc. Together they generate the sense of a body or physical self. Moreno generally describes psychodramatic roles as imaginary roles that may be fantastic, such as the role of the ghost or alien. Any role that one can imagine oneself taking or that one longs to embody falls under this category. Moreno is not consistent in classifying roles that are acted out in life. In some of his writings, these seem to be social roles but sometimes he considers them to psychodramatic. Psychodramatic roles are the basis of that which we call the psyche. The social roles are conserves and are similar to the roles in a drama in that they prescribe the behavior of the members of society who are taking them. The social roles produce that which we call society.

Moreno distinguishes between role playing, role taking, and role creating. Childhood creative play is the model for role playing. Children spontaneously play house, school, cops and robbers, and other roles as they try to make sense of the society into which they have been born. *"Playing a role is the personification of other forms of existence through the medium of play.* It is a *specialized* form of play …" (J. L. Moreno, Z. T. Moreno & Moreno, J. D., 1955, p. 108). All of psychodrama and sociodrama involves role playing. Role taking is embodying an established role like a role in a play in conventional theater or a social role. Here the role conserve serves as a constraint on those who take, limiting their freedom. Role creating occurs by placing individuals in situations which are unlike any with which they are familiar. There is a high degree of freedom in role creating. This was the primary mode of Moreno's original spontaneity theater and is a part of today's improvisational theater.

Some form of role playing almost always precedes role taking. Role training, which Moreno introduced at the Hudson Training School, is the most systematic approach, allowing one to experiment with the role long before taking it. Role training has been widely used in business and industrial settings. Politicians have learned to use the method before press conferences and debates. Another form of role playing is rehearsal. Many people who find themselves called upon to be in the role of a public speaker give their speeches to one or two others, or to no one, several times before they give the one that counts. There is also the mental role training that many individuals conduct before entering a new situation, a rehearsal in one's imagination.

Psychodrama is a systematized method of role playing. Past events that were puzzling or painful are enacted in an attempt to restore emotional equilibrium. Current pressing problems are explored in search of a path to follow. Anticipations of the future are produced to serve as guidance. All are accomplished through role playing and the techniques of psychodrama.

Tele

> Tele is defined as a feeling process projected into space and time in which one, two, or more persons may participate. It is an experience of some real factor in the other person and not a subjective fiction. It is rather an inter-personal experience and not the affect of a single person.
>
> *(J. L. Moreno, 1946, p. 238–239)*

It is a very common experience. We find ourselves thinking about someone who is important to us but with whom we have been out of touch., perhaps deciding that we should give that person a call or send an email. The phone rings and who is calling but the one about whom we have been thinking. Most of us have had or know someone who has had the experience of having an intuition that a relative or close friend has died, often being waked in the night with a strong sense of the event. Coincidence? Conventional psychological science has no other reasonable explanation. For Moreno, it is an example of telic communication.

Tele is a two way sensitivity that people have for each other, a communication that occurs at a distance, hence the name. When we first meet another person, we immediately have some idea of who they are and a positive feeling drawing us toward them, a negative feeling pulling us away from them, or a neutral feeling, neither attraction or rejection. Interaction with the other can confirm or correct the initial impression. An initial neutral reaction may become positive or negative; a positive perception first impression may become negative or a negative one may become positive. However, initial impressions tend to have considerable validity.

Two other processes related to tele are transference and empathy and Moreno used them to help define tele. Transference, a concept introduced by Sigmund Freud, is a reaction to another based on that person's resemblance to someone we already know. It differs from tele in that it is a one way process and involves a distortion of the other person. With interaction over time, Moreno stated, transference diminishes as tele increases. Empathy, originally brought to bear on the psychology of aesthetics by German psychologist, Theodore Lipps, is a process of sensing the feelings of another person. Although it shares validity with tele, it is, like transference, a one way process. Tele involves reciprocity. It also has the quality of non-locality as evidenced when your friend in San Francisco about whom you have been thinking calls you in New York. Non-locality is a quality that is incompatible with classical physics although it appears in quantum physics.

The phenomenon of tele suggests that we know more about others than we usually give ourselves credit. Scientific skepticism is widespread in a society that values rationality as highly as our society does and we are cautioned against intuition and first impressions: "Don't judge a book by its cover" or "Looks are deceiving," for example. This may be reasonable advice but experience tells us that intuitions can also be trustworthy.

Telic phenomena are often identified in psychodrama sessions. Psychodrama groups are made up of people who have not previously met. In a psychodrama, the protagonist is frequently asked to select a member of the group to serve as an auxiliary ego, that is to represent an absent person from the protagonist's social atom, perhaps a family member. At the end of the drama and in sharing with the protagonist, it is not unusual for the auxiliary to say something like, "I don't know why you picked me for that role, but I have had the same kind of experience that person had." It is also common that members of the group anticipate being selected to become an auxiliary. A frequent statement heard during sharing is "I knew you were going to pick me to be your mother (father, sister, brother, uncle, etc.)"

When any group of people assembles there is a lot of communication occurring. Members of the group who previously knew each other greet and exchange words. Those who are strangers may or may not introduce themselves to each other. Many feelings are stirred up, both positive and negative and are flowing through the group. We have feelings of attraction and rejection. These emotions have a significant impact upon the ensuing actions of the group, often serving to warm up various members to the issues and problems they are struggling to resolve. We often identify a psychodrama by the protagonist's name because it is the life experience of this person that provides the content of the drama. However, in more ways than one every psychodrama is the psychodrama of the group that produces it. Everyone is involved in what happens, in direct and very subtle ways.

Emotion

J. L. Moreno did not present a detailed theory of emotion although emotion is very much a part of sociometry and psychodrama. Psychodramatists, however, learn a lot about emotional life. I have found that a theory presented by Joseph De Rivera (1977) describes emotional phenomena very much as I have encountered them in psychodrama, and I have found it extremely helpful in understanding and dealing with emotions psychodramatically. The word emotion is derived from the Latin *mover*, to move out, and De Rivera's theory is based on phenomenological research on the movement of emotions, that is to say, how emotions underlie our actions. This makes the theory especially applicable to a phenomenological method based on acting out.

Emotions are intentional, meaning that an emotional response always has an object. It is a response to something perceived. One is not simply angry; one is angry at something, an individual, a thing, an event, or some situation. De Rivera considers emotions as instructions which tell the individual how to behave in the present situation. The movement is not simply a reaction to a stimulus but rather a transaction, a rearrangement between oneself and the object of the emotion experienced.

The transformation may be an alteration of the distance between self and object for example. There are four possible transformations involving distance between self and object:

Reducing distance between self and object:

Self moves toward object.
Object is moved toward self.

Increasing distance between self and object:

Self moves away from object.
Object is moved away from self.

Each of these movements is characteristic of an emotion. Love, for example, instructs the self to reduce distance between self and object by moving oneself toward the object. Desire, on the other hand, instructs the self to reduce distance by moving the object of the emotion toward oneself, to possess it. Fear instructs one to increase distance by moving oneself away from the object, while anger is an instruction to move the object, a barrier between the oneself and one's goal, away from oneself.

There are a number of emotions in which the object of the emotion is not an other but oneself, anxiety, depression, security, and confidence, for example. De Rivera recognizes that these would not qualify as emotions in some theories. Since they involve transformations, he includes them. "Even calmness," he claims,

> the antithesis of what many would call an emotion, is considered an emotion, provided that calmness does not refer to some affectless state, but rather to the implicit transformation involved when a person is calm in spite of a demanding situation.
>
> *(p. 45)*

De Rivera sees the four emotions mentioned above, anxiety, depression, security, and confidence as counterparts to the belonging emotions, fear, anger, love, and desire. He provides a rationale, not necessary for this discussion, to explain the relationships. However, many other writers in the fields of psychotherapy and emotions have noted a relationship between anxiety and fear, and between anger and depression. The movement and instruction of these emotions are the factors relevant to psychodrama. The movement of the emotion, security, is allowing the world to come into the self, and the instruction is "Let go." This is demonstrated by the secure child who can let go of the parents hand and explore the surroundings. The movement of confidence is expanding the self into the world, and the instruction is "Take hold." The confident person does not relinquish his or her position in the face of opposition. A very important principle of emotion is that when an instruction of an emotion has been successfully completed, the original emotion will dissipate and be replaced by another. Another way of saying that is that when an emotion has been sufficiently expressed, it will yield to other emotions.

Important emotions for the psychodramatic psychotherapist are anxiety and depression, both of which are considered pathological when they approach a high intensity. The movement of depression is constricting, moving the self away from the world and the instruction is "Give up." The movement of anxiety is keeping the world out of the self and the instruction is "Hang on" to one's self.

Emotion can be considered as the initial evaluation of the situation in which one finds oneself. When an individual perceives a threat to one's physical self the emotional response is fear and the instruction of fear is "Get away from it." Conversely, if a protagonist experiences fear, the director knows that the protagonist perceives a threat to the self. When, on the other hand, one perceives an obstacle or barrier blocking one's path to a desired goal, one experiences anger and the instruction is "Get it out of the way." If an individual is angry but doesn't know why, a condition with which the psychodrama director sometimes must deal, a search for something standing between the individual and a goal can be conducted.

Depression is the response to loss and the instruction of depression, "Give up," informs the person experiencing it that a wound has occurred and that they need time and space to heal and relinquish that which has been lost. A situation in which something threatens the psychological integrity of the individual results in anxiety and hence its instruction, "Hang on" leads to a defending posture. Understanding emotion in this way can be of great assistance to the psychodrama director.

Catharsis

Sigmund Freud introduced the term, catharsis, into psychiatry by referring to the cathartic method of Joseph Breuer, his co-author of *Studies in Hysteria* (Breuer & Freud, 1895/1982). When Dr. Breuer's patient, now famous as Anna O., was in a hypnotic trance, she would re-experience the original event associated with one of her many hysterical symptoms. The symptom would subsequently disappear. Freud called this response abreaction. He was initially convinced that the cathartic method was a cure for hysteria. However, when he found that the symptoms returned after a period of time, he gave up both catharsis and hypnosis in favor of free association.

Freud very likely thought of catharsis as purging, a common interpretation of catharsis. in this case as a purging of emotions which he believed to be the by-product of frustrated id impulses. He may have been influenced by Anna O's description of the process as chimney sweeping. There is, however, another way to understand the concept which was employed by Aristotle in his writings on both medicine and the theater. In Aristotle's time, medicine was based on the notion of humors, an imbalance of which resulted in disease. His use of catharsis, then, may have meant a rebalancing of the humors. When Aristotle hypothesized that watching the ancient Greek tragedy resulted in a *katharsis* of pity and fear for the audience, Moreno suggested that he meant "a kind of homeopathic relief from their own selfish passions" (J. L. Moreno, 1940a, p. 209).

While endorsing Aristotle's hypothesis about the effect of the theater on the audience, Moreno reasoned that there must be an even greater catharsis from actually taking the role of a character in a tragedy. The actor's catharsis was the basic principle in his first endeavor in the use of spontaneity theater techniques to ameliorate psychological problems. In addition to distinguishing between audience catharsis and the actor's catharsis, Moreno made a distinction between abreactive catharsis and integrative catharsis. Finally, he distinguished between action catharsis and intellectual or cognitive catharsis.

Abreactive Catharsis

Abreaction is a sudden and intense expression of emotion associated with an event from the past, an expression that was blocked or suppressed at the time it was aroused. It is not uncommon, for example, for children to suppress anger at or fear of their parents in moments of heated interaction between them. In many cultures or subcultures, expression of certain emotions is routinely discouraged. Boys, for example, may be pressured to suppress fear. Adults, too, find many situations in which discretion calls for not revealing what one is feeling, especially when one is confronting powerful authorities who can affect one's future.

Abreaction is the process described by Freud and is catharsis as it is ordinarily regarded in the field of psychotherapy. Although Freud gave up the cathartic method, other psychoanalytic theorists, like Wilhelm Reich (1949) and a number of the nonpsychoanalytic psychotherapies, such as Janov's primal scream (1970), Casriel's new identity therapy (1972), and Lowen's bioenergetics, (1976) claimed abreactive catharsis to be therapeutic. These methods tended to subscribe to a hydraulic theory of emotion. In this conceptualization, emotions were considered to be entities that if blocked of expression could build up pressure and seek release in other ways. Catharsis was the discharge of the built up tension and provided relief to the individual (Nichols & Efran, 1985).

Abreaction occurs frequently in psychodrama, probably more so than with non-action methods of psychotherapy. This is due to the fact that the whole person is involved in psychodrama, not just the cognitive components. Abreaction is a function of memory and, as psychodramatists have long known and neurological researchers have recently discovered, memory is a neuromuscular process, not merely a neurological one. Although abreactive catharsis occurs often in psychodrama, especially with protagonists who are new to the method, abreaction is not a goal that the experienced director seeks. Instead it occurs spontaneously and unexpectedly to the protagonist. Abreaction has a dramatic impact on the audience and the protagonist, and a significant skill for the psychodrama director to learn is to be comfortable with intense displays of emotion. Although abreaction is not a goal of psychodrama exploration, it does serve a purpose in facilitating catharsis of integration.

Catharsis of Integration

Mental catharsis is here defined as a process which accompanies every type of learning, not only a finding of resolution from conflict, but also of realization of self, not only release and relief but also equilibrium and peace. It is not a catharsis of abreaction but a *catharsis of integration* (J. L. Moreno, 1953, p. 546).

The life events that protagonists present for psychodramatic exploration often fall into one of several familiar categories. They are situations in which interpersonal transactions have been unsuccessful, in which the protagonist has been betrayed, emotionally hurt, or traumatized, in which an act or action has been blocked, or which have left the protagonist puzzled by the way in which a transaction has gone. They also include occasions that have left the protagonist experiencing guilt, regrets, or anxiety. When they are remembered, the emotion associated with these experiences is also recalled in full force. The catharsis of integration alleviates the pain of emotional wounds and allows protagonists to regain their power from those who have taken it away, brings understanding to the mysteries of why significant others have acted in certain ways, and allows the protagonist to complete the blocked act. Integration may also allow for the assuaging of guilt and resolution of regret.

Integration is accomplished in psychodrama by virtue of the flexibility of surplus reality to slow events down and speed events up as the protagonist may need. Thus events that happened in a few minutes can be expanded and explored at leisure. Events that may be separated by years in time but intimately linked by emotion and meaning can be experienced in the space of minutes in psychodrama. All the techniques of psychodrama are designed to explore at depth the genuine feelings of protagonists as well as those of the significant others who share time, space, and living with them. Role reversal, soliloquy, the double and the safety of the psychodrama stage allow the protagonists to perceive situations from the point of view of the significant other, from a deeper self perspective free of the evasion and inhibition they may feel in real life, and, through the psychodramatic mirror, to view the situation from outside it, a more objective point of view.

Catharsis of integration is also achieved by confronting those toward whom the protagonist may feel guilt and exploring the circumstances that allowed or forced the protagonist to violate his or her own ethical standards. This is particularly helpful for protagonists when the significant other is no longer in their lives. Protagonists report a sense of a great burden being relieved by an encounter with a deceased parent with whom the protagonist had unresolved issues at the time of the parent's death. Catharsis of integration is often the completion of unfinished business.

Everyone, Moreno said, craves to embody far more roles than those we are allowed in everyday life. We have our official roles with their expectations, responsibilities, and privileges but we imagine ourselves in others. A stock broker may daydream of being an acclaimed artist, a school teacher wishes she were a paleontologist. These psychodramatic roles in various degrees of development create tensions and anxiety as the constraints of life restrict us to official roles. Moreno often utilized this notion in psychodramatic therapy, especially but not exclusively with psychotic patients. In an article on his treatment of 33 schizophrenic, bi-polar, and depressed patients, Moreno (1940b) describes in detail how allowing psychotic patients to live out their fantastic inner worlds with the help of auxiliaries on the psychodramatic stage can bring their imaginary worlds "into an equilibrium with the official reality so that [they] might be able to live in the open community without harm to anyone and without any frustrations of [their] own aspirations" (p. 130). Moreno applied this principle in his early treatment of the marital problems of one of his spontaneity players, described in an earlier chapter of this book. This particular approach to the catharsis of integration is not widely used by today's psychodramatists.

Action Catharsis vs. Insight

Moreno contrasted action catharsis with intellectual catharsis or insight. Insight, defined as gaining a new understanding of one's behavior or actions, is the goal of many methods of psychotherapy in which dialogue is the primary modality of communication. Experiencing a reorganization of one's perception of the situation is qualitatively different from an intellectual understanding or ability to explain one's behaviour (Cornyetz, 1947). The experience seems to affect every fiber of the individual's being and has significantly more powerful impact. Many individuals who have had extensive psychotherapy report that in their initial experience as a protagonist they *feel* for the first time all the insight that they have gained in psychotherapy. Psychodrama has been called the method for people who have more insight than they know what to do with.

Interpersonal versus Individual Psychotherapy

Physical illness and diseases are situated in the afflicted individual and the individual is the focus of treatment. Even though there are efforts to control the spread of contagious infections, treatment is still treatment of the infected individuals. The principle that pathology belonged to the individual was carried over when emotional disturbances became the purview of psychiatry, a medical category. Psychiatry became the treatment of individuals with emotional problems and these problems were categorized as psychopathology.

J. L. Moreno, although himself a doctor and a psychiatrist, saw things differently. He considered most of the phenomena of psychopathology to be the products of interpersonal relationships. His viewpoint is quite clearly seen in an article entitled "Interpersonal Therapy and the Psychopathology of Interpersonal Relations" (J. L. Moreno, 1937). Here he relates the story of his treatment of three interlocked people, each of whom exhibited symptoms of a serious nature. The first person involved in treatment was a wife who complained that her husband had lost interest in her and was having an affair with another woman. "She suffered from hysterical attacks, suicidal ideas, and insomnia". She disappeared from time to time but then always returned home. These symptoms had stymied the husband's desire to leave her to be with his lover. She made it clear that what she wanted was for her husband would give up the other woman and return his affections to her. If he did so, Moreno was convinced, the wife's symptoms would disappear. At the wife's request he contacted the husband to see if this was feasible. He discovered that the husband was experiencing serious emotional distress as well. His ability to work had suffered to such a degree that he was afraid of losing his job. He had made an attempt at suicide. He was preoccupied with thoughts of how many people would be hurt if he were to carry through on his desire to kill himself. He suffered from depression. Also, he no longer loved his wife or wanted to stay with her. Finally, again at the wife's request, Moreno met with the "other woman," the woman with whom the husband had fallen in love. This woman, too, was adversely affected by the situation. She was fearful that harm might come to her and her brothers because of the affair. She had become socially withdrawn to the point of being agoraphobic and she was depressed.

Moreno continued to meet with all three people involved in the triangle, individually and in various combinations. He assisted them in more fully expressing their respective positions to each other. and in understanding the positions of each other. Over time, the wife came to accept that the relationship with her husband would not improve. The two mutually agreed to a divorce. The husband the other woman eventually married.

Taken individually, each member of the triangle had symptoms that would warrant psychiatric treatment. By the standards of psychoanalysis, the primary method of psychotherapy of the time, no practitioner would have agreed to see more than one member of the three. Each might have been in individual analysis for a very long time. Moreno perceived the situation very differently. Instead of three persons with individual neuroses, he recognized three people presenting an interpersonal neurosis. His sociometric work as well as his psychiatric experience led him to believe that all psychiatric problems involved interpersonal relations.

Moreno addressed psychosis as the disruption of normal interpersonal interactions in his therapeutic approach to treatment of psychoses (J. L. Moreno, 1940b). At the time, psychosis was widely considered to be a psychological phenomenon. The notion of the schizophrenogenic mother was a prevailing concept in the mental health field. Moreno was prescient in believing that the psychoses had a significant constitutional component, a common position today.

At about the same time that Moreno was developing sociometry and psychodrama, psychoanalysts were beginning to consider social effects upon personality development and psychopathology. Karen Horney, Erik Erikson, and especially Harry S. Sullivan (1953), (who coined the term, interpersonal psychiatry, were among the theorists who established what became known as social psychiatry. Even though this expansion of psychiatry greatly expanded the psychoanalyst's total concentration upon the individual, Moreno was disdainful of it. Social psychiatry does indeed pay attention to the effect that social factors have upon the development of personality, especially the development of mental structures likely to foster psychiatric symptoms. Moreno's objection was that social psychiatry, as does biomedical psychiatry, continues to see pathology as residing within the individual. The individual remains the focus of treatment.

Moreno envisioned a new science that he called sociatry. "The world is full of isolated, rejected, rejecting, unreciprocated, and neglected individuals and groups" (1953, p. 118), he wrote. His viewpoint was that the social health of humankind depends upon attacking the pathology of normal groups. To do so is the aim of sociatry. Psychiatry treats the individual psyche and soma. Sociatry treats the pathological syndromes of normal society, of inter-related individuals and inter-related groups. It is based on two hypotheses: 1) "The whole of human society develops in accord with definite laws"; 2) "A truly therapeutic procedure cannot have less an objective than the whole of mankind" (p. 119)

Moreno described sociatry as remedial sociometry. It includes all the instruments of sociometry, the sociometric experiment, role testing, spontaneity testing, role training, and psychodrama. Moreno predicted that a profession of sociatry would be established in the future. Sociatry would not be restricted to practitioners of medicine as was psychiatry. Rather, it would include those now in the fields of education, psychology, and sociology. It would be established on the knowledge contributed by all social and psychiatric sciences. In anticipation, Moreno accepted as students for training in sociometry and psychodrama all who came seeking to learn about his theories and methods.

The Triadic System

"I merged group psychotherapy, sociometry and psychodrama into a single system: the Triadic System. The triadic system is the integration of three theories: the science of the group, the science of sociometry and the science of action. These are interrelated and indispensable to one another" (J. L. Moreno, 1964, p. 156).

Group Psychotherapy

In "Open Letter to Group Psychotherapists," Moreno (1947) lectures group psychotherapists on the differences between group psychotherapy and individual psychotherapy. The patient in individual psychotherapy is an individual *person*, Moreno says, and any method of psychotherapy is based on a knowledge of the structures and dynamics of the individual *psyche*. Group psychotherapy is the therapy of a group of individuals with the emphasis placed on *group*. Group therapy is based on a knowledge and understanding of the structure and dynamics of the *group*. Moreno goes to great lengths to point out that there is a substantial difference between the concepts applicable to individual psychotherapy and those germane to group therapy, and that groups cannot be understood by projecting the concepts of individual psychotherapy upon them. He assails psychoanalytic group therapists as major violators of this principle. Rather than projecting such concepts as hysteria or the Oedipus complex upon the group, he insisted, the group therapist must deal with the organization of the group, the positions of the individuals comprising the group, the psychological currents within it, and the attractions and rejections existing between the group members.

The basic idea, common to all true group psychotherapies, is that the interactions of individuals in groups can be therapeutic. This leads to the basic rule of group therapy: every individual the therapeutic agent of the other individual; every group the therapeutic agent of the other group. The therapeutic power no longer resides in the group therapist whose task is to find ways for group members to help each other.

In a later article, Moreno (1951) made a shorter and more direct argument against employment of concepts from individual psychoanalysis in group therapy. At least call it psychoanalysis in a group setting, he pled, and leave the term group psychotherapy to those who invented it. He emphasized the dependence of group therapy on sociometry as well as the relationship of group therapy with action methods such as psychodrama. "There is hardly a session without "psychodramatic episodes" (there is no stage required for them) between patients, between patients and their relatives, between patients and therapists" (p. 283).

Sociometry, Science of the Group

Sociometry is J. L. Moreno's theory that there is a hidden structure underlying the official organization of every group. This structure consists of the attractions and rejections that group members have for each other with respect to the specific activities in which the group engages. Sociometry provides a method for revealing that structure as well as for reorganizing groups to promote optimal functioning. Finally, sociometry is a method of social research and has yielded a number of principles regarding social structure. These include the sociogenetic law, the sociodynamic law, and basic types of leadership.

Moreno maintained that sociometry provided the science that underlay group psychotherapy and psychodrama. The sociometric configurations in a group, such as positive and negative stars, pairs, chains and others, certainly account for much of what happens in a group, whether it is a therapy group or a different type of group. A group leader is at a great advantage in knowing these structures and how they function. The group itself can benefit from the revelation of its hidden sociometric structure. None the less, some writers, e.g. Kellermann (1992), believe that a knowledge of sociometry is unnecessary to the practice of psychodrama, and many of today's practitioners have at best a rudimentary grasp of the sociometric method. Few psychodramatists make greater use of sociometry beyond selection of protagonists and the action social atom (Seabourne, 1963). Action continua (or spectrograms), methods to reveal group information, are sometimes considered to be sociometry. While they can be quite helpful, they are, at best, quasi-sociometric instruments. Ann Hale has been the foremost advocate for sociometry for several decades, has written extensively on sociometric topics (Hale, 1985, 2012; Hale & Little, 2005), and created the International Sociometric Training Network located at: www.sociometry.net. A wealth of information is available on this website to anyone interested in sociometry and psychodrama. This includes over 40 articles that can be accessed for free.

Here is an example of how sociometry is helpful to a psychodrama training group. There were nine participants in a psychodrama training group which was part way through a weeklong training workshop. The trainer, Jack, became concerned because one member of the group, Harry, was receiving an over-abundance of negative attention from other members of the group. He knew that this was detracting from the potential learning experience for the group. He proposed that the group undertake a sociometric exploration to learn about the sociometric method and to better understand the interrelationships within their group. There was some initial resistance from several group members but two who had previous experience with sociometric exploration helped convince the reluctant ones that it would be a positive experience.

1. Jack discussed the importance of criteria, that a criterion must be a specific activity and that the activity should be one in which the group can expect to engage. The members chose two:
2. With whom do I choose to spend half an hour in a psychodrama doubling exercise?
3. Who in this group do I choose to direct me in a personal psychodrama?

Simple forms similar to those devised for the purpose by Hale (1985) were passed out for each criterion, and the group members made three lists of their fellow trainees: positive choices; rejections or "negative" choices; and neutrals, neither chosen nor rejected. The group had agreed in advance to make all information generated available to the whole group. After they had completed the paperwork, each member spent a few minutes with each other member, discussing the choice they had given and the reason they had made that choice.

The choices from the separate forms were entered into a sociomatrix. The sociomatrix for the criterion of choosing a director is depicted in Figure 7.2. The names of the group members are written in the spaces provided along the left side of the form and, in the same order, along the top. The rows across show choices made. The columns reflect choices received. Thus, we can see that Suzie gave Jack first choice, Lyle second, Marcia third, Alice fourth, and Robyn fifth choice. Harry received her first and only negative choice, and she neither chose nor rejected Judith. That is called a neutral.

	Suzie	Judith	Alice	Marcia	Robyn	Carolyn	Lyle	Harry	Jack		Positive Made	Negative Made	Neutrals	
Suzie			4	3	5		2	-1	1		5	1	2	
Judith	5		1	3	6	-1	4		2		6	1	1	
Alice		-3		1		3	-2	-1	2		3	3	2	
Marcia	-2		1		3	4		-1	2		4	2	2	
Robyn	7	6	3	2		4	5		1		7	0	1	
Carolyn	5		2		3		4	-1	1		5	1	2	
Lyle	3	-2	2	1				-1			3	2	3	
Harry	1	4	-3	-4	3	2	-2		-1		4	4	0	
Jack	5		2	1	4	3		-1			5	3	0	
											42	17	13	
Positive Received	6	2	7	6	6	5	4	0	6		42			
Negative Received	1	2	1	1	0	1	2	6	1		15			
Neutral Received	1	3	0	1	2	2	2	2	1		14			
Positive Mutuals	3	1	3	3	5	3	1	0	5		24			
Negative Mutuals	0	1	1	0	0	0	2	4	1		9			
Neutral Mutuals	0	0	0	0	0	0	0	0	0		0			

FIGURE 7.2 Sociomatrix

Reading downward, we can see that in return, Suzie received a first choice from Harry, third choice from Lyle, fifth choices from Judith, Carolyn, and Jack, and a seventh from Robyn. In addition to displaying all choices made and received by group members, the sociomatrix has a place for showing the total number of choices made and received by each group member as well as mutual choices. All these numbers have meaning for the sociometrist and help explain interactions in the group that may otherwise seem puzzling or unusual. For example, Judith received relatively few positive responses and three negative. On the other hand, she makes six positive and one negative choice. A group leader can anticipate that she wants to be better accepted in the group than she is. The group leader will want to help her ameliorate her sociometric position, perhaps by encounters with those who gave her negative choices. Lyle is in a slightly less vulnerable position but the leader will look for ways of helping him find ways to improve his sociometric position.

A sociogram was constructed from the results of the sociometric test. It is reproduced in Figure 7.3. Moreno liked to use red lines to indicate positive choice and black ones for negative choice or rejection. However, sociograms can be produced monochromatically by utilizing solid and dotted or dashed lines as in this case where a solid line indicates positive choice and a dotted line is used for rejection. There are multiple ways of drawing sociograms. In these examples, first choices are shown. If

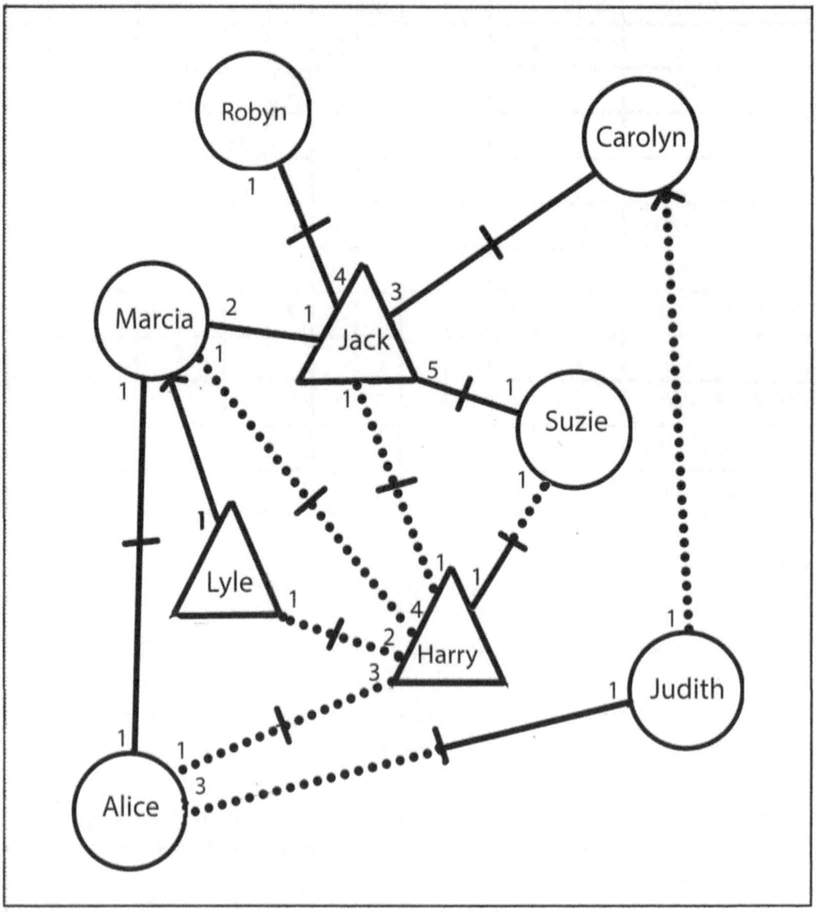

FIGURE 7.3 Group Sociogram

a first choice is reciprocated by any level response, that is also shown. The small numbers near the circles (females) and triangles (males) indicate the level.

Sociomatrices and sociograms show the same data. Each is superior in certain ways. The sociogram gives a holistic picture of the group; the sociomatrix is better for counting choices, choices made, choices received, mutual choices and the like. A sociogram can also be constructed for each individual. Figure 7.4 is one that shows choices made and received for Harry.

Harry, of course, is the problem child of the group, a fact which everybody, including Harry himself, recognized even before the sociometric exploration. He is clearly a negative star in this group. He receives six rejections, all first negative choice, and gives more negative choices than anybody else. He is in danger of becoming a group scapegoat or even extruded from the group. He has managed to alienate most of the members, including the trainer, Jack, who has made efforts to alleviate his estranged position. Not only is Harry an irritation in the group but

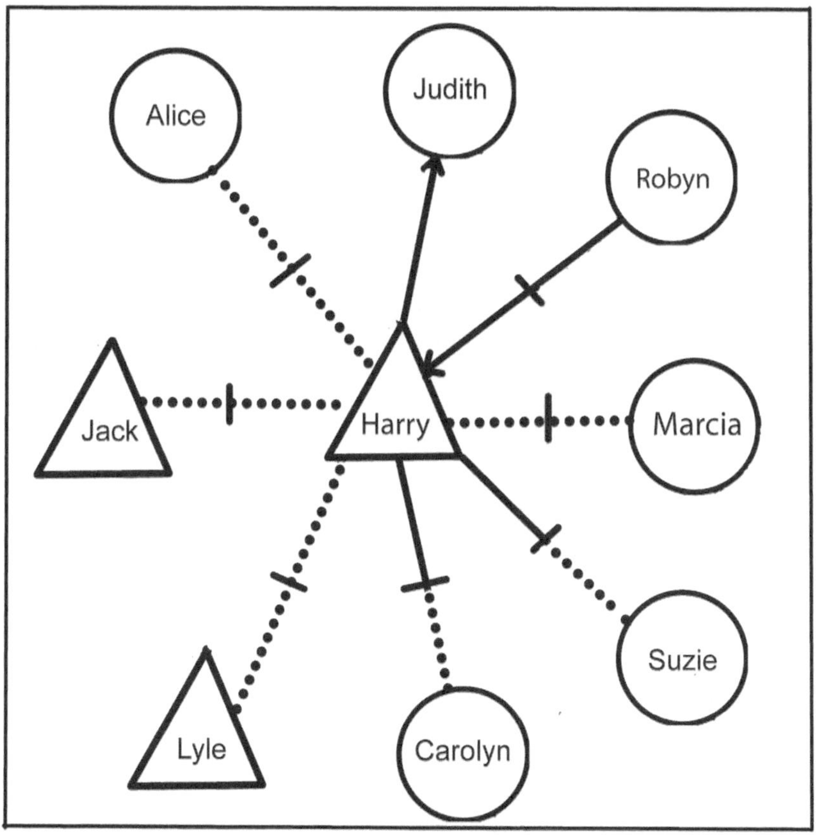

FIGURE 7.4 Harry's Sociogram

Jack believes that he, like every other group member, has something in terms of life experience to contribute to the group. Until his sociometric position is improved, it is likely that his contributions will be rejected by the group.

After the sociometric test had been completed and group members had shared with each other the reasons for their positive and negative choices, the group discussed their experiences of sociometric exploration. There was general agreement that it was hard work to assess feelings accurately and then to report them honestly. This was especially true of rejections. At the same time, several group members said, it was a positive thing to learn how people felt about each other. Judith reported that it was a relief to deal with the negative choices she received. She had felt the rejection and talking with those individuals had been helpful. Both Judith and the members who gave her negative choices felt that something had been cleared up and all felt closer to each other.

Harry was an exception. He knew before the sociometry, he said, how people felt about him and that he would get a lot of rejections. Jack asked him if it were common for him to be rejected in groups. He replied that he wasn't much of a group person and more of a loner. In school, he tended to be liked by teachers more than by classmates. A graduate student in chemistry, he had signed up for the psychodrama workshop at the recommendation of a counselor who thought it would be a helpful experience for him. In reality, he had felt uncomfortable and in a strange world from the minute the workshop began.

"Would you like to take a look at why that is happening to you?" Jack asked. Harry agreed. Jack asked the group how they felt about Harry being the next protagonist. All thought it would be a good idea and after a break, Harry's psychodrama began.

The formal sociometric experiment takes a lot of time to carry out. It would be excessively unwieldy for even a relatively small group to attempt formal sociometry for every activity it undertakes. However, experience with the full sociometric experiment gives one an extremely valuable way of looking at groups, a kind of a template, so to speak. The effects of personal choice and rejection are influencing the actions of every group; sociometry only makes them visible.

Psychodrama

Psychodrama, sociodrama and all the variations are the third leg of the triadic system. Since this book is aimed at explicating the psychodramatic method, little else needs to be added here.

Note

1 There are echoes here of Moreno's first publication, *Ein Ladung zu Einer Begegnung (Invitation to an Encounter)*, in which Moreno first points to the problems and dangers of over valuing the conserve, especially the cultural, or manmade, conserve. From

Moreno's perspective, it would have been much better to meet Sorokin in person and discuss their ideas about spontaneity and creativity than to write and send articles to each other.

References

Bergson, H. & Mitchell, A. (1911/1944). *Creative evolution*. New York: Random House.

Bohm, D. (1980). *Wholeness and the implicate order*. London: Routledge & Kegan Paul.

Breuer, J. & Freud, S. (1895/1982). *Studies in hysteria*. New York: Basic Books.

Casriel, D. (1972). *A scream away from happiness*. New York: Grosset & Dunlap.

Cornyetz, P. (1947). Action catharsis and intensive psychotherapy. *Sociatry*, 1, 59–63.

De Rivera, J. (1977). *A structural theory of the emotions*. New York: International Universities Press.

Hale, A. & Little, D. (2005). *Sociometric processing of action events*, revised ed. Toronto: Toronto Centre for Psychodrama and Sociometry.

Hale, A. E. (1985). *Conducting clinical sociometric explorations: A manual for psychodramatists and sociometrists*. Roanoke, VA: Royal Publishing Company.

Hale, A. (2012). *Three cyclical models which enhance consciousness of interpersonal connection*. Roanoke, VA: VA International Sociometry Training Network.

Janov, A. (1970). *The primal scream*. New York: Dell.

Kellermann, P. (1992). *Focus on psychodrama: The therapeutic aspects of psychodrama*. London: Jessica Kingsley.

Kipper, D. A. (1967). Spontaneity and the warming up process in a new light. *Group Psychotherapy*, 20, 62–73.

Lowen, A. (1976). *Bioenergetics*. New York: Penguin Putnam.

Moreno, J. L. (1937). Inter-personal therapy and the psychopathology of inter-personal relations. *Sociometry*, 1, 9–76.

Moreno, J. L. (1940a). Mental Catharsis and the Psychodrama. *Sociometry*, 3, 209–244.

Moreno, J. L. (1940b). Psychodramatic treatment of psychosis. *Sociometry*, 3, 115–132.

Moreno, J. L. (1946). *Psychodrama volume 1*. Beacon, NY: Beacon House.

Moreno, J. L. (1947). Open letter to group psychotherapists. *Sociatry*, 1, 16–30. Reprinted in J. L. Moreno, in association with A. Friedemann, R. Battegay, & Z. T. Moreno (Eds.) *The international handbook of group psychotherapy*. New York: Philosophical Library. 17–22.

Moreno, J. L. (1951). The situation for group psychotherapy. *Group Psychotherapy*, 3, 281–283.

Moreno, J. L. (1953). *Who shall survive?* Beacon, NY: Beacon House.

Moreno, J. L. (1955a). Canon of creativity. *Sociometry*, 18, 359–360.

Moreno, J. L. (1955b). System of spontaneity-creativity-conserve, a reply to P. Sorokin. *Sociometry*, 18, 382–392.

Moreno, J. L. (1955c). The discovery of the spontaneous man. *Group Psychotherapy*, 8, 103–129.

Moreno, J. L. (1955d). The significance of the therapeutic format and the place of acting out in psychotherapy. *Group Psychotherapy*, 8, 7–19.

Moreno, J. L. (1955e). Theory of spontaneity-creativity. *Sociometry*, 18, 361–374.

Moreno, J. L. (1956). The dilemma of existentialism, Daseinanalyse and the psychodrama with special emphasis upon "existential validation. *International Journal of Sociometry and Sociatry*, 1, 59–60.

Moreno, J. L. (1960a). Discussion of Ehrenwald's dialogue "psychoanalyst vs psychodramatist." *Group Psychotherapy*, 13, 74–75.

Moreno, J. L. (1960b). Role. In J. L. Moreno et al (eds.). *The sociometry reader*. Beacon, NY: Beacon House. 80–86.

Moreno, J. L. (1961). The role concept, a bridge between psychiatry and sociology. *The American Journal of Psychiatry*, 118, 518–523.

Moreno, J. L. (1964). The third psychiatric revolution and the scope of psychodrama. *Group Psychotherapy*, 17, 149–171.

Moreno, J. L. (1965). Therapeutic vehicles and the concept of surplus reality. *Group Psychotherapy*, 18, 211–216.

Moreno, J. L. (1989). The autobiography of J. L. Moreno, M. D. (Abridged). *Group Psychotherapy, Psychodrama & Sociometry*, 42, 3–52.

Moreno, J. L. & Moreno, F. B. (1944). Spontaneity theory of child development. *Sociometry*, 7, 89–128.

Moreno, J. L., Moreno, Z. T. & Moreno, J. D. (1955). The discovery of the spontaneous man. *Group Psychotherapy*, 8, 103–109.

Moreno, Z. T., Blomkvist, L. & Reutzel, T. (2000). *Psychodrama, surplus reality and the art of healing*. London/New York: Routledge.

Nichols, M. P. & Efran, J. S. (1985). Catharsis in psychotherapy: A new perspective. *Psychotherapy*, 22, 46–58.

Nolte, J. (2014). *The philosophy, theory and methods of J. L. Moreno*. New York: Routledge.

Reich, W. (1949). *Character-analysis*. New York: Noonday Press.

Seabourne, B. (1963). The action sociogram. *Group Psychotherapy and Psychodrama*, 16, 145-165.

Sorokin, P. (1955). Remarks on J. L. Moreno's "theory of spontaneity-creativity". *Sociometry*, 18, 118–126.

Sullivan, H. S. (1953). *The interpersonal theory of psychiatry*. New York: W.W. Norton.

Thurber, J. (1939, March 18). The secret life of Walter Mitty. *The New Yorker Magazine*.

8

A BRIEF HISTORY OF PSYCHODRAMA

J. L. Moreno, who is also the originator of sociometry, and is one of several "fathers" of group psychotherapy, is universally credited with originating the psychodrama method. Moreno discussed the origin of the psychodramatic method at some length in the opening pages of his book entitled *Psychodrama, First Volume* (1946). He apologized for the references to his life experiences in the discussion but notes that the method was created out of his experiences in conducting groups of many kinds in many places. The theory came later. Understanding how it developed, he hoped, would throw light upon its nature.

Search for the King of Austria

The first official psychodramatic session, Moreno stated, took place in a theater, the *Komodienhaus*, in Vienna, on April 1, 1921. Vienna was a city, at the time, of great unrest and instability, a result of World War I. Vienna had been the capital city of the Austro-Hungarian Empire which had broken up into a number of individual states as a result of the war. Vienna's reason for existence had disappeared with the Empire. Moreno set out to "treat and purge the audience from a disease, a pathological cultural syndrome which the participants shared. Postwar Vienna was seething with revolt. It had no stable government, no emperor, no king, no leader" (1946, p. 1).

The theater was full that night. A huge crowd, diplomats, representatives of government, and of religious, political, and cultural organizations was in attendance. This was not surprising because it had been announced that the new king of Austria would be in attendance. That announcement certainly was designed to draw a crowd. Seven o'clock came. The curtain went up—on a stage empty except for a large, red plush, high backed, gilded, armchair, a throne for the new king. Moreno appeared on the stage. He introduced himself as the king's jester. "But where is the king?" he asked. "It was announced that he would be here. He is not on the stage so he must be in the audience." For the next three hours, he conducted tryouts for the role of the king, the role of leader of the country. He invited the members of the audience to come to the stage, sit on the throne and act like a king. The audience was to judge the performance. At the end, nobody passed the test. None were found worthy of being the king and Vienna remained leaderless.

Although every student of Moreno learns that this event was the first psychodrama, it was more of a sociodrama, psychodrama's sister method that deals with the social roles rather than individual roles. At the same time, the search for the king also could be considered the first role training exercise. The affair caused quite a stir. The Viennese press was quite disturbed by the incident. Moreno wrote that he lost many friends and in his journal, noted *"nemo profeta in patria* (never a prophet in one's own country)" (1946, p. 2).

The Young God Player

In the same pages that he describes the search for the King of Austria, Moreno tells another story that has become a feature in the lore of psychodrama. I would be remiss not to include it here. When Moreno was somewhere between four and a half and five years old, he and neighborhood children were playing in the basement of his parent's house while the parents were out visiting. Little Jacob suggests that they play God, offering to take the title role while the other children could be his angels. They placed chairs on a huge oak table, tying them together, and then piled more chairs on top, making several layers until they reached the ceiling. The children helped Jacob climb up to and sit on the top chair while they circled around the table as angels, using their arms to fly. "Why don't you fly?" he was asked. He tried it, stretching out his arms, and quickly ended up on the floor with a broken arm. "This was," he wrote, "as far as I can recall, the first 'private' psychodrama I ever conducted. I was the director and subject in one" (1946, p. 2). Moreno referred to the incident as the Psychodrama of the Fallen God. He learned, he said, that even God needs helpers, and sometimes described psychodrama as therapy for fallen gods.

The concept of God and especially of God-as-creator was a preoccupation for Moreno, and figures into all his philosophy, theories, and methods. Moreno mused that the layers of heavens up to the ceiling may have been the first inspiration for the many levels of the psychodrama stage. He gradually learned, Moreno wrote, that other children liked to play God also.

For about three years, just before and just after he matriculated at the University of Vienna, Moreno established himself as the Mysterious Story Teller of the *Augarten*, the public park that surrounded the palace of the Emperor. He showed up always wearing a long green cloak and entertained the children he found playing there by telling them fairy tales. Imaginative, the stories were always new. He engaged the children in creating them and in spontaneous play. It was, he wrote, a crusade for children to have their own society and rights, rejecting established social stereotypes. He permitted them to play God when they wanted to and when they fell short, "I began to treat children's problems by letting them act spontaneously" (1946, p. 3). Parents and teachers prevailed upon him to conduct a children's theater. One of the children for whom he was a tutor was Elisabeth Bergner who grew up to become one of the most popular and successful stage and screen actresses in pre-World War I Germany.

Das *Stegreiftheater*

Regardless of the parts that the incident of the broken arm played in the development of psychodrama, as well as the Search for the King of Austria, the next major step in the evolution of psychodrama was the establishment of the *Stegreiftheater* (Marineau, 1989; J. L. Moreno, 1989). In 1921, Moreno joined a group of actors who met regularly at Café Museum in Vienna. The group included actors Alexander Moissi, Hans Rodenberg, Robert Blum, Robert Grunwald, and Ladislaus Lowenberg (renamed Peter Lorre by Moreno) as well as Anna Höllering whose father owned the Komodienhaus theater and had loaned it to Moreno for the Search for the King. Elisabeth Bergner joined them when she was available. Some writers, Robert Müller, George Kulka, Franz Werfel, and Fritz Lampl also belonged to the group. They were all involved in the Search for the King episode. A preoccupation of the group was how to make theater more relevant in the turbulent society of post-war Vienna.

Moreno conceived the idea for the *Stegreiftheater*, a theater of spontaneity. He proposed going back to the very first Ancient Greek dramas that were spontaneously created religious rites instead of written dramas. His spontaneous theater would be a purer form of drama. In the conventional theater (Moreno called it the "conserve" theater), he said, all the creativity is hidden. It takes place behind the scenes. The playwright conceives the play alone in his study. The theatrical company assigns the roles to actors, and the director rehearses them in private. All the audience sees is the final product. In the conventional theater, the actors are separated from the audience to enhance the illusion of reality. In the theater of spontaneity, on the other hand, the actors take, perform and create their roles simultaneously. There is no playwright, no rehearsal, minimal props and scenery, and no backstage to hide things. The creativity is all in the open, available to the spectators who are no longer passive watchers but who take part in the proceedings.

Under Moreno's direction the group spent a year training and searching for a theater. They found it at Maysedergasse 2, a large room that could seat 40 or 50 people. Here, the group spontaneously produced dramas with themes suggested by audience members, from the actors themselves, or from ideas given by Moreno, the director. Reviewed by the theater critics of the local newspapers, the *Stegreiftheater* gained a reputation. The small theater was full every evening. A problem quickly arose. Accustomed to the conventional theater and to social stereotypes in their lives and in the theater, the audiences mistrusted spontaneity. They suspected that the spontaneously created dramas of the *Stegreiftheater* were rehearsed—unless a scene went badly. In that case they were convinced that spontaneity theater didn't work. To deal with this obstacle, the Stegreiftheater company devised the living newspaper. They collected the latest editions of the Viennese newspapers and enacted the news stories from them. Obviously, there was not time to have scripted and rehearsed these dramas. They had to be spontaneously created as advertised.

Resolving a Marital Problem

At some moment, during the several years that the *Stegreiftheater* was in operation, an event took place that was a major advance toward development of the psychodramatic method. An actress who was often assigned the ingénue roles, playing the part of the endearingly innocent and wholesome, artless young woman and a young writer became enamored, eventually marrying. In writing about the event, Moreno calls the actor Barbara and the young writer George. One day not long after the marriage, George came to Moreno asking for help. Unless things changed, he said, the marriage would fail. The problem was that when she was alone with him, she was the opposite of the roles she played on stage. She was abusive, used profane words, and would even strike George with her fists. Moreno promised to see what he could do. That evening when she came to the theater, Moreno talked to her. He told her that he was afraid that the audience might tire of seeing her always in the same roles and that he thought it might be well for her to try some roles in which she would portray

> the rawness of human nature, its vulgarity and stupidity, its cynical reality, people not only as they are, but worse than they are, people as they are when they are driven to extremes by unusual circumstances. Do you want to try?
>
> *(p. 4)*

She did want to try and was enthused by the idea. In the news that day was a report of the murder of a prostitute by an *apache*, a Parisian gangster type, in the red light district. Barbara was assigned the role of the prostitute. In the first scene the prostitute and apache come out of a café. They get into an argument. She wants more money. The argument turns violent. Barbara becomes a hellcat. She swears at the man and kicks him repeatedly in the leg. The *apache* gets violent. He pulls out a knife and starts chasing her. It becomes so realistic that the audience thinks that the actors have lost control. Some members stand up and shout "Stop! Stop!" The apache finally catches her and stabs her to death.

Afterwards, Barbara was quite excited. From then on, she was assigned low life roles, barmaids, gun molls, revengeful wives, and jealous girlfriends. George reported that things were changing at home. Although she still started arguments, they were less heated and did not last so long. George also reported that watching her play these new roles on the stage affected him also. He was more tolerant and less impatient with Barbara.

Moreno then suggested that Barbara and George play scenes together on the stage. They played scenes that resembled those in their daily life and, later, scenes from their original families. Audience members, Moreno wrote, often told him how deeply the Barbara–George dramas touched them, more deeply than the other dramas the troupe presented. After some months, Moreno discussed with the two marriage partners the development of their psychodrama, analyzing each of the sessions with them.

The principles that Moreno called upon to resolve the troubles in the Barbara–George marriage are unique to psychodrama and to Moreno's role theory. First is his notion that all of us fantasize or daydream about roles in which we would like to act but which the course of our lives does not give us an opportunity to do so. Elements of these wished-for roles sometimes seek expression through roles that we take in everyday life. For Barbara, we can speculate that social pressures were in the way of her being a shrew and expressing angry, violent feelings, at least in public. At the same time, she apparently received much approval and admiration for her ingénue roles, both on and off stage. The unexpressed feelings can create great inner tensions. In the intimacy and privacy of her relationship with her husband, she relieved this tension by being a virago, picking fights where she could scream and curse at him freely. George had no counter-role with which to adequately engage with her in this situation. By giving her roles in which she could express this part of herself on the stage, Moreno reduced the tensions that led to the behavior threatening her marriage.

As always, Moreno saw disruptive or disturbing behavior as interpersonal rather than contained within the individual, and the resolution of such behavior is achieved by dealing with the individual's social atom.[1] This was the reason for involving George in the process. By acting out their interactions on the spontaneity stage George and Barbara gained a better understanding of each other. The dramas in which they revealed to each other important events from their families of origin deepened these insights and led to greater tolerance for each other.

The psychodramatic method as we know it today evolved gradually over a long period of time, incorporating many events. The Barbara and George marriage was not the only use of dramatic techniques in which Moreno engaged during this period of his life. In his biography of Moreno, Marineau (1989) informs us that

Moreno assisted another couple, Robert and Diora, explore their marriage on the *Stegreiftheater* stage. Working with families, Moreno used an approach that he called *theatre reciproque* that employed acting techniques. Marineau also refers to Moreno's treatment of a suicidal man, a story that I heard from Martin Haskell, one of the outstanding figures in the psychodrama collective during the 1950s through the 1990s. A young man came to Moreno asking for assistance in committing suicide. Moreno had a number or sessions with him and listened to his tale of how he had made mistakes at every turn and now his life was so messed up that it was no longer worth living. Moreno finally suggested that since he had bungled everything else in his life maybe he should rehearse his suicide so that he didn't botch that also.

They set the scene. The patient took a psychodramatically lethal dose of medicine. After he had died psychodramatically, Moreno pointed out that there was a problem. They now had a body and had to deal with that. A funeral was in order. The young man agreed. Another scene was set, a church. The patient described it and indicated where the coffin would be located. Moreno than had him identify who would be present for the occasion, and had him reverse roles with each person he named. He then laid in his coffin. Moreno then asked him, "Is there anybody here that you would like to talk to?" The young man thought about it and replied that yes, he would like to talk to his father.

"It's too bad that you are dead," Moreno pointed out. "If you are dead, you can't talk to your father. However, you can talk to him if you choose life. Which shall it be, life or death?" The young man chose life.

Psychodrama thus developed step by step. Moreno emphasized the fact that he had tried out his ideas before writing about them, the opposite of philosophers whom he disdained for presenting beautiful theories in their writings while leaving it up to politicians and others to implement them. He had applied his methods in a variety of situations before he was presented them to the world.

Immigration to America

The next events from which psychodrama unfolded took place in the United States where Moreno had immigrated in December, 1925. The first year or two were not easy, according to Marineau. Moreno apparently worked on a device for magnetic recording, co-invented by Franz Lörnitzo and himself. He had a temporary visa that he managed to get renewed by traveling to Canada. At some point, he met Dr. Bela Shick, a pediatrician at Mt. Sinai Hospital and the inventor of the famous Shick test. Through the good offices of Shick, Moreno conducted some spontaneity work with children. He also worked with Shick on spectroanalysis for a while. He also met Beatrice Beecher, granddaughter of famous preacher, Henry Ward Beecher. She worked at the Plymouth Institute of Brooklyn, and invited Moreno to demonstrate his methods there. Learning of his visa difficulties, she offered to marry Moreno so that he could become a citizen of the United States. Moreno took her up on the offer and they were married in 1928, and by the original agreement, divorced in 1934. In 1927, he took the examination to be licensed as a physician in New York State.

Moreno met William H. Bridge, professor of public speaking at Hunter College, when giving demonstrations of spontaneity techniques at different schools and colleges. Bridge was supportive of Moreno's desire to try the spontaneity theater in America and suggested the name Impromptu in lieu of spontaneity theater. Moreno recruited a group of players, trained them and began holding three sessions a week in a rented studio of Carnegie Hall.

He also founded a journal called *Impromptu* at the same time, "to interpret and elaborate a philosophy of the creator as an anti-mechanical corrective to our age" (J. L. Moreno, 1931, p. 3), and to present the technique of Impromptu theater. He published several short discussions of various aspects of his philosophy of spontaneity–creativity as well as the text of an Impromptu drama and a description of an Impromptu test. Other contributions to the journal included a favorable review by drama critic A. B. W. Smith (1931), and an article on the spontaneity drama by Viennese author, Robert Müller (1931). J. J. Robins (1931a, 1931b,) author, editor, poet, stage director, teacher of theater and one-time assistant to Constantin Stravinsky (Archives and Manuscripts, n.d.), had articles in both issues of *Impromptu*.

In between dramas, Moreno invited members of the audience to take an "Impromptu Test." Moreno later called this a spontaneity test. A volunteer was invited to take the stage and a scene that Moreno would provide was set. As the individual entered the scene, Moreno would introduce a factor that required the volunteer to act. In one example, he told the volunteer that a fire had started in the house, that there was a baby in one room and valuable jewels in another. As the volunteer dealt with the situation, Moreno tossed in other problems: for example, a relative was about to walk into the house just under the room that was on fire and it might crash in on her. After the test, Moreno would offer an analysis of the individual's performance.

Moreno used a variety of spontaneity techniques in his work with the students of the New York State Training School for Girls at Hudson where he conducted his first sociometric study of an entire community. He made use of spontaneity and situation tests to assist in determining where girls should be placed in the community. He also employed role training to prepare students for their return to open society. He directed psychodramas here for psychotherapeutic purposes as well.

Beacon Hill Sanitarium

The systematic development of the psychotherapeutic function of psychodrama began after Moreno bought an estate in Beacon, NY, and established Beacon Hill Sanitarium in 1936. He built the first psychodrama theater in the carriage house of the property and began the psychodramatic treatment both with outpatients and patients admitted to the Sanitarium. He soon developed a reputation for his successful treatment of schizophrenic patients. This was particularly notable because the primary psychotherapy at that time was psychoanalysis and Freud had declared that schizophrenic individuals could not be psychoanalyzed. Psychiatrists in the area began referring psychotic people to Moreno for treatment.

The psychodrama method evolved. Initially, Moreno worked with patients in the theater one at a time. He would take the individual, or the couple if he was conducting marital therapy, and one or more staff members to play auxiliary roles into the theater where he would direct the psychodramatic work. He discovered that psychotic patients had a particular sensitivity to each other and could benefit from observing and participating in each other's dramas. Moreno began working with groups of patients.

In the early years of psychodrama, after a reenactment, Moreno would talk with the protagonist and analyze what had happened on stage. One day he worked with a patient in front of a group of professional mental health professionals. After the action session, the group became very busy analyzing the material. Moreno noticed the protagonist becoming more and more uncomfortable. The positive impact of the psychodrama was rapidly seeping away. He stopped the analyzing. He directed the professionals to start talking about their own experiences, how their personal life events were related to those of the protagonist. He insisted that they share rather than analyze (Z. T. Moreno, 2006, p. 22). To this day the post-action phase of the psychodrama session has shifted from analysis to sharing.

As late as the early 1940s, an assumption was widely held that nobody but Moreno had the ability to direct a psychodrama. Psychodramatic psychotherapy was not considered a learnable method. This notion may have been augmented by Moreno's work with schizophrenic patients. Moreno was unusually successful with these severely disturbed people, perhaps more so than anyone else. It may be that no one ever conducted psychodramatic psychotherapy as successfully as Moreno although others have employed psychodrama with psychotic patients. Jim Enneis at St. Elizabeth Hospital in Washington, D.C., certainly did so, and I conducted psychodrama groups with patients who were diagnosed as psychotic at the Fulton State Hospital #1 in Missouri. Moreno, however, seemed to have a unique ability to relate to these individuals. Zerka used to say that Moreno "could talk schizophrenia."

Zerka Toeman Moreno

Zerka Toeman came to Beacon Hill Sanitarium in 1942, and became an essential factor in the continuing development of the psychodramatic method. When Zerka became part of the staff of the sanitarium, she, too, subscribed to the belief that only Moreno could direct a psychodrama. In her autobiography, she wrote that she never dreamed of directing psychodrama and had no ambition to do so. Her desire was to be the best double possible. This was important because Moreno used double egos extensively in his work with schizophrenic patients. Zerka, as she had wished, became Moreno's favorite auxiliary ego (Z. T. Moreno, 2006, 2012).

Eventually, she was encouraged by Moreno to take the directorial role. Over the years, Zerka developed her own distinctive style. When Moreno directed a psychodrama, it tended to be heavily focused on interrelationships in the protagonist's current social atom. Dramatizations of the protagonist's past experiences were certainly not absent in his directing but they played a less important role in his overall conduct of therapy than did current relationships. Zerka, on the other hand, tended to put more weight on the impact of previous experiences in the protagonist's current life difficulties. In her autobiography, *To Dream Again*, Zerka (2012) speculates that Moreno's emphasis upon the current situation may have to do with his desire to distance psychodrama from psychoanalysis and its heavy emphasis upon the past. I think his priority of the present was also motivated by his fascination with the complexity of role relationships and by the importance he placed on living in the here and now.

As Moreno grew older, he relied more and more on Zerka to direct the demonstrations in hospitals and universities, which the Morenos conducted all over the country. She also took on increasing responsibility for training as Beacon Hill Sanitarium became the Moreno Institute and emphasized training over treatment. After Moreno's death in 1974, Zerka kept the Moreno Institute in operation for some years. She also traveled internationally, giving demonstrations and conducting training workshops in many countries. She continued actively training into her nineties, passing away in 2018. Now, 40 years after Moreno's death, more currently active psychodramatists, myself included, have been influenced by Zerka Moreno's style of directing than by J. L. Moreno's style.

The Classic Version of Psychodrama

Moreno (1953) described the classic type of psychodrama in Preludes of the Sociometric Movement:

> First of all, it was entirely spontaneous. The spontaneity of the group was as important as the spontaneity of the director. It was unrehearsed and more even than this, it was entirely unplanned and there was, for me, also a fundamental reason for "not" planning it. It was to be here and now and not yesterday or tomorrow. I did not want to see or know anything about the people in advance, so as to keep all my own and their spontaneity free for the moment of meeting. It was to be a meeting at first sight.
>
> *(p. 71)*

The life events, fantasies, dreams, or anticipations of future events of one individual, the protagonist, became the material upon which the drama was based. He also said that the drama was co-produced by the protagonist and the director, the protagonist furnishing the content and the director providing the techniques by which the content was turned into action on the stage.

Moreno realized that every director, even though trained by him, would develop a unique individual style of directing. This was a recognition that psychodrama is an art form, a dramaturgy. Just as the pictures of the same barn, painted by the members of an art class will be different from each the other, reflecting the individual way of seeing and using the painter's instruments, a psychodrama will reflect the personal style of the director. A classic drama directed by one person would look different if another had directed it. However, just as the barn will be recognizable in the various pictures made by the class, protagonists will be perceived for who they are, regardless of who directed the psychodrama.

Until the establishment of the Board of Examiners in Psychodrama, Sociometry and Group Psychotherapy in 1974, every certified psychodramatist had been trained at least in part at the Moreno Institute. Training at the Institute served as a standard, the state of the art, so to speak. This feature of psychodrama training no longer existed when people could be certified without having a common training experience. Training at the Moreno Institute imparted a far greater standardization of practice than does the Board of Examiner's examination and demonstration of skills. As a result, there is now much greater diversity in the training and practice of psychodrama. This diversification grows with each succeeding generation of trainers.

Note

1 This is similar to the current practice of some family therapists and the concept of identified patient. This is usually a child whose disruptive behavior has brought family into treatment. The disruptive behavior is considered the signal of dysfunction in the family social system.

References

Archives and Manuscripts (n.d.). *J. J. Robins Papers*. New York: The New York Public Library.

Marineau, R. (1989). *Jacob Levy Moreno, 1889–1974*. New York: Routledge.

Moreno, J. L. (1931). Editorials. *Impromptu*, 1(1), 3.

Moreno, J. L. (1946). *Psychodrama, First Volume*. Beacon, NY: Beacon House.

Moreno, J. L. (1953). Preludes of the sociometric movement. In J. L. Moreno. *Who Shall Survive?* Beacon, NY: Beacon House. 13–108.

Moreno, J. L. (1989). The autobiography of J. L. Moreno, M. D. (Abridged) Part 2. *Group Psychotherapy, Psychodrama & Sociometry*, 42, 59–125.

Moreno, Z. T. (2006). *The Quintessential Zerka* (edited by T. Horvatin, E. Schreiber). New York: Routledge.
Moreno, Z. T. (2012). *To Dream Again.* Catskill, NY: Mental Health Resources.
Müller, R. (1931). The Impromtu theater in Vienna. *Impromptu*, 1, 14–15.
Robins, J. J. (1931a). Impromptu for America. *Impromptu*, 1(1), 23–25.
Robins, J. J. (1931b). The poet in Impromptu. *Impromptu*, 1(2), 6.
Smith, A. (1931). The Impromptu theater in New York. *Impromptu*, 1, 5–7.

9

THE ASPIRATIONS OF J. L. MORENO

Jacob L. Moreno was a far more remarkable person than many who have been endowed with greater fame. It is not that he, and especially his psychodramatic method, are not widely known; psychodrama is practiced on all the inhabitable continents. However, Moreno faced rejection and derision by his psychiatric colleagues during his most productive years. The theories and instruments that he gave to sociologists and social scientists were often badly used or even misused with respects to the purposes for which they were created. His sociometric ideas still have not been fully exploited. At the same time, most of his innovations have entered the mainstream of psychotherapeutic practice.

Moreno famously told Sigmund Freud, "You analyze people's dreams. I intend to teach them to dream again." Moreno himself had enormous dreams, far more expansive than creating a new method of psychotherapy. His true ambition was recorded in the first sentence of his major opus: "A truly therapeutic procedure cannot have less an objective than the whole of mankind" (J. L. Moreno, 1953b, p. 3). He aspired to bring that therapeutic procedure into being.

God Playing

In his autobiography, Moreno (1989a) said that his fascination with God began at an early age. "The most famous person in the universe was God and I liked to be connected to Him" (p. 19).

The childhood God playing event in which he broke his arm, reported in the previous chapter, was only one of the many God playing games of that he organized with playmates, according to his biographer (Marineau, 1989). He took up God playing again in early manhood, at about the time he began interacting with children in the gardens of Vienna. J. L. Moreno's son, Jonathan, has suggested Moreno's God playing was something of a mind experiment, the kind of exercise that Albert Einstein popularized. Moreno sometimes referred to what he did as role reversal with God. I have listened to Moreno talk about his God playing and I think it quite possible that Jonathan is correct and that J. L. Moreno gave himself an assignment something like: What if I were God and decided to come to earth as a human being myself instead of sending my Son. What would I do as a human being to make things better when confronted with poverty, hardship, and injustice?"

The God playing period lasted through the experience, which resulted in the publication of *Des Testament des Vaters* (1920), translated later by Moreno as *The Words of the Father.* This was an occasion during which Moreno heard God's words, an occurrence described in some detail by both Moreno (1989b) and Marineau (1989). This work, as many writers including his biographer, expresses Moreno's philosophy and theology, and contains many concepts that later appear in his scientific work. Morenean exponents are divided with respect to this work. Some think it is inspired and others are embarrassed by it. Moreno's references to playing God and encouraging others to also do the same, was the source of much derision and criticism by many of his psychiatrist colleagues in the early days of psychodrama. Moreno's detractors pointed to *The Words of the Father* as evidence that Moreno was mentally unstable, even psychotic. Imagine, however, that everyone in the world reversed roles with the God of responsibility and creativity as described in *The Words of the Father* at the same time. Moreno said that all the inspirations for his later work came from the period of God playing.

"The Vienna of 1910," Moreno claimed,

> was one of the display grounds of the three forms of materialism that have since become the undisputed master of our age, the economic materialism of Marx, the psychological materialism of Freud, and the technological materialism of the steamboat, the airplane, and the atomic bomb.
>
> *(1947b, p. 5)*

All were deterministic and rejected the notion of spontaneity. Many writers, including Sigmund Freud, had noted that humanity had endured a number of cosmic blows over a few hundred years. Copernicus demonstrated that Earth, the home of humankind, was not the center of the universe. Darwin showed humans to belong to biological evolution. Marx showed history to be determined by mass movements, not individuals. Freud claimed that man acted from unconscious drives instead of his will. Moreno (1947b) concluded that, "A careful analysis of Man's total situation has made clear to us that the process of his secularization of his religious, social and cultural institutions has developed too fast" (p. 10).

A New Form of Religion

Marxism and psychoanalysis both rejected religion. Moreno chose a different approach. He contended that a new sort of religion, a positive religion, should be tried. This was a religion that would incorporate in its inspirations and techniques, insights from science, including some from Marx and Freud:

> My position was threefold: first, the hypothesis of spontaneity-creativity as a propelling force in human progress, beyond and independent from libido and socio-economic motives—which does not deny the fact that they are frequently interwoven, but which does deny the contention that they are merely a function and a derivative; second, the hypothesis of having faith in our fellowmen's intentions—outside of obedience resulting from physical and legalistic coercion—the hypothesis of love and mutual sharing as a powerful, indispensable working principle in group life; and third, the hypothesis of a superdynamic community based upon these principles which can be brought to realization through newer techniques. It may be said that *I tried to do through sociometry what "religion without science" has failed to accomplish in the past and what "science without religion" has failed to accomplish in Soviet Russia.*
>
> *(1953a, p. 14)*

Creativity, which has had a connection with the divine from the muses of Greek mythology to the Creator God of monotheism was the centerpiece of Moreno's undertaking. Moreno undertook a scientific study of creativity. The *Stegreiftheater* was his laboratory. His theory of spontaneity and creativity, and the connection between the two, crystallized during the time of his engagement with children in the gardens of Vienna. He concluded that spontaneity, which he described as deviation from the laws of nature as well as the matrix of creativity, was the necessary catalyst for creativity to become manifest at all levels of being, physical, biological, sociological, psychological, and spiritual. Most importantly was the fact that spontaneity was trainable.

The Theater of Spontaneity

Moreno's first attempt at introducing the public to the importance of spontaneity was *Das Stegreiftheater*, from 1922 until about 1925. Creativity on the spur of the moment was the promise of the "theater of spontaneity which opened its gates to the worshipers of immediate creative genius" (J. L. Moreno, 1947b, p. 6). He anticipated that people would find spontaneous drama more honest and compelling than the conventional theater and that the theater of spontaneity would be a serious competitor. He quickly discovered that his new theater faced huge difficulties from the audience. They had been brought up to distrust their own spontaneity in favor of relying on cultural conserves.

> Therefore when true spontaneity was presented to them in the Stegreiftheater either they suspected it to be well rehearsed and an attempt to fool them, or, if a scene was poorly played they considered that as a sign that spontaneity does not work.
>
> *(p. 7)*

Encountering the same response in both Europe and America, Moreno turned his energies in other directions. None the less, the theater had provided a laboratory for the systematic study of spontaneity–creativity phenomena. The ground was prepared for the emergence of psychodrama.

Group Psychotherapy

The opportunity to test his ideas about therapeutic interaction came with his appointment in 1931 to develop a classification system for prison inmates of Sing Sing Federal Prison. This resulted in the publication *Application of the Group Method to Classification* (J. L. Moreno, 1932). Although the classification method that Moreno and his faithful assistant, Helen Jennings, devised was complicated and never adopted (Jennings, 1943), the paper gave Moreno a chance to promulgate his basic ideas on group therapy. *Application of the Group Method to Classification* was republished with additional material as *The First Book on Group Psychotherapy* (3rd Ed.) (1957).

Convinced that the major source of emotional disequilibrium lay in relationships between people rather than residing in the individual, Moreno pioneered marital, family, and group methods. It was not until psychiatric casualties of World War II overwhelmed the capacity for individual psychotherapy that group therapy became acceptable to the psychiatric community. Although Moreno's reputation as a group therapist brought him recognition and an opportunity to demonstrate his methods, his major principle, that the healing power lay in the group rather than in the therapist, was and continues to be largely neglected. Most of the activity, other than psychodrama, that goes under the label of group therapy is what Moreno called "individual psychotherapy in a group setting" (1947a). Therapeutic interaction among group members, the healing power of the group, however, occurs even in the groups where it is not recognized by the group therapist.

Sociometry

The Sing Sing Prison project led to Moreno's 1932 appointment as Director of Research at the New York Training School for Girls at Hudson, the site of his foundational sociometric research. Publication of *Who Shall Survive?* (1934), a report of his work at the School, stirred up immense excitement and enthusiastic interest in sociograms and sociometric questionnaires among sociologists and social psychologists. Two decades of research inspired by sociometry, thousands of articles according to Hare and Hare (1996), followed. Only a few of the authors understood that Moreno considered sociometry to be an action method and that a sociometric experiment was not complete until the group in which it was carried out had been re-organized along the choices made by its members. Researchers excited about sociometry produced articles on reliability and validity as well as ways of presenting the data and methods of analyzing it instead of exploring group phenomena like social networks. Rather than using the data from the sociometric test to therapeutically re-organize groups, researchers correlated the results with other kinds of test measures, subverting sociometry from the task for which it had been created.

After publishing *Sociometry*, the journal he had founded to report sociometric research, for 18 years, Moreno gave it to the American Sociological Society. Moreno (1955) wrote an eight-page article giving a number of reasons for this action. He did not say so but I have long suspected that he tired of the resistance of sociologists and social psychologists to employ sociometry in the way for which he had devised it, and, as with spontaneity theater, he gave it away.

Psychodrama

It was psychodrama, the lifeboat for spontaneity theater, that turned out to be the method which kept Moreno's aspirations alive after he decided that resistance to the spontaneity theater was too great to overcome. Psychodrama has perhaps suffered less from the separation of method and theory than sociometry and group psychotherapy, but suffer it has. French psychoanalyst Serge Libovici (1956) practiced psychoanalytic psychodrama enactment, apparently as early as 1947. After enacting a scene, in which auxiliaries were prohibited from exercising their spontaneity, the director would interpret the material with respect to resistance and transference. Since then, other therapists have combined psychodrama with many non-Morenean theories, an anathema to Moreno. Based on a reductionist philosophical basis they provide a personality theory, a structured framework from which to understand the client's behavior. These theories impose limits for understanding behavior compared to accepting it at face value.

It is my opinion that many psychodramatists trained in recent decades are more timid than those of us who were trained at or in the ethos of the Moreno Institute. Asked what the most important personal characteristic a psychodramatist needs, Moreno did not hesitate. "Courage," he said. The director needs courage to take the protagonist into and through the deepest, darkest thoughts, fantasies, fears, and events that the protagonist has suffered. To be a courageous director, one needs to explore his or her own emotional life thoroughly as a protagonist in order that emotional problems and inhibitions won't impede his or her directing of another.

One of several possible explanations of the erosion of psychodrama is that a large majority of those who become trained psychodrama directors enter training after having been educated and socialized as psychotherapists. They have learned theories of personality, psychopathology, and been introduced to methods of psychotherapy. These theories are based on the conventional scientific foundation of reductionist, positivist philosophy, and scientific materialism. They view the psychodrama method from the perspective of the conventional psychotherapist. Despite these tendencies, the basic techniques of psychodrama have been sufficiently retained that much of the power of psychodrama has survived.

When lawyers began attending psychodrama training workshops, I observed that they often learned to direct more rapidly than did mental health professionals. When I paid a visit to Zerka Moreno after working with lawyers for several years, I mentioned that observation to her. "That's because they don't have so much to unlearn," she said without hesitation. That had been my surmise also.

Psychodrama is so different from other methods of psychotherapy, even those like Gestalt Therapy or Transactional Analysis, which were inspired by psychodrama, that I have come the conclusion that psychodrama can be more accurately described as an *alternative* to psychotherapy than as a *method* of psychotherapy. That idea is based on several considerations.

Psychotherapy literally means treatment of the mind. Psychotherapy is widely practiced in accord with the medical model of psychotherapy, described by Wampold (2001) as having five components: client disorder, problem or complaint; a psychological explanation for the problem; a mechanism of change; therapeutic ingredients that are specific for the disorder, problem, or complaint. Pressures to practice within this framework come from psychiatry's hegemony in the field of mental health, including its authoritative *Diagnostic and Statistical Manual of Mental Disorders* (2015), as well as insurance companies who pay for psychotherapy. Psychodrama does not require diagnosis or a psychological explanation for the client's problem or even a theory of psychopathology. When a man walked into Moreno's office, proclaiming to be Adolf Hitler, Moreno did not conduct a psychiatric examination, record a diagnosis, or prescribe a treatment plan. Nor did he bother to point out the absurdity of the man's claim. Instead, Moreno took the man to the psychodrama theater stage balcony and invited him to address his subjects, students waiting to hear from Moreno. Psychodrama is holistic while the medical model is atomistic or fragmentary. Psychodrama techniques may individually be helpful to the protagonist, but it is the session as a whole, including warm up, action, and sharing that make a difference in the protagonist's life.

Psychodrama differs from all so-called talk psychotherapies by putting the client on his or her feet and into action. What a director does is markedly different from that of a conventional psychotherapist. Psychodrama differs from other experiential therapies in that the action is modeled after life and takes place in the controlled surplus reality of the psychodrama stage. Psychodrama engages the whole person with all his or her thinking, remembering, emoting, and acting. It is truly holistic.

Psychotherapy is based on the notion that a malfunction exists and that the task of therapy is to repair or restore. Psychodrama is based on the idea that one has not learned correctly from one or more of one's life experiences. Psychodrama gives the protagonist the opportunity to re-experience an event in a controlled setting to extract a more effective meaning from it. Psychodrama has an existential, phenomenal philosophical basis. Psychotherapeutic methods are typically founded in conventional scientific positivist, reductionist philosophy. Psychotherapy is a treatment method; psychodrama is an educational method.

Moreno vs Freud

Moreno must have been surprised to find how widely accepted psychoanalysis was in the psychiatric community. That had certainly not been so in Vienna where people avoided even mentioning Freud's name. His opportunity to demonstrate his negative judgment of psychoanalysis came at the first Annual Conference of the American Psychiatric Association that Moreno attended, in 1931. Much to his surprise, he was invited to comment on the presidential address that Abraham Brill gave to American Psychoanalytic Association, holding its own conference conjointly with the APA. Brill presented a psychoanalysis of Abraham Lincoln whom he diagnosed as schizoid-depressive. Moreno began his comments by stating that "It was not fair to psychoanalyze the personality of a man now dead, as you have to do it without his consent" (1953a, p. 45). He criticized Brill for using statements of friends and contemporaries for his material, people who were not professionals. He suggested that Brill's choice of an illustrious, outstanding character such as Lincoln, revealed more about Brill's unconscious psychodynamics than it did about his subject. Moreno's assault on psychoanalysis was reported in the next morning's newspapers, earning him a degree of fame. However, it also undoubtedly generated antipathy from psychoanalysts, perhaps a majority of his psychiatrist colleagues.

Moreno's feud with psychoanalysis and Sigmund Freud has been routinely interpreted as envy of Freud's greater fame. Moreno must have regarded the prestige of psychoanalysis with some degree of despair, recognizing the tremendous resistance that it would present to his concepts of spontaneity and creativity. However, his enmity, which was actually greater to analytic theory than to Freud, was directed at the psychological materialism of psychoanalysis which held that psychological phenomena could be reduced to biological precepts. Particularly inimical to Moreno's spontaneity-creativity was the idea of creativity as the sublimation of libido, sexual energy. Perhaps Moreno's most scathing comment on Freud was this passage:

> Freud looked at man from below; he saw man "upside down" and from the position from which he looked at man he saw first his sexual organs and his rear. He was profoundly impressed, perhaps oversensitized, and he never turned his attention away from them. But one can evaluate

man more advantageously by looking at him from above. Then one sees him erect, standing on his feet, eyes and head first.

(1953a, p. 53)

Trenchant perhaps, but descriptive of how Moreno perceived the difference between them. Moreno could even be complementary toward Freud, describing him as an excellent clinician and a better scientist than many of his detractors. Moreno's criticisms were not very different from the recent spate of anti-Freudian literature.

Why Isn't Psychodrama Better Known?

None of the 48 lawyers in the first class of the Trial Lawyers College had any previous experience with psychodrama. After three days of psychodramatic personal growth work, many of them asked why psychodrama wasn't more widely known. Their most common guess was that psychodrama was so effective that the psychotherapy profession had suppressed it for economic reasons! I wish that was not so distant from the truth.

Several explanations have been offered to account for psychodrama's position on the margin of psychotherapy. Moreno himself proclaimed "There is no controversy about my ideas, they are universally accepted. I am the controversy" (1953a, p. 108). Controversial though he was in many ways and to many people, I don't accept this statement as valid, and I suspect he did not either. Haskell (Borgatta, Boguslaw & Haskell, 1976) was more accurate when he wrote that Moreno and his work were the subject of controversy because he challenged so many established concepts in psychiatry, psychology, and sociology. In my opinion, Boguslaw in the same article was exactly right when he said, "Moreno's most profound contributions were always destined for marginality in a society whose central ethos revolves about industrial production and its concomitant rationalization of everyday life" (p. 156).

Moreno acknowledged that he had failed to accomplish what he had set out to do. Certainly society seems to have gotten even more materialistic since Moreno considered it potentially destructive to humanness. At the same time, as Jonathan Moreno (1989) writes, "the force of Moreno's creative genius was such that his ideas penetrated the society, even if his reputation remained marginal, appreciated mostly by those in the know" (p. 10). We have yet to appreciate a superdynamic community of humankind based on the principles of spontaneity–creativity, love, and mutual sharing. None the less, Moreno did create methods which have the potential for nudging us toward the creation of such a world. It remains for them to be employed in the way Moreno intended.

References

American Psychiatric Association (2015). *Diagnostic and statistical manual of mental disorders*. Arlington, VA: American Psychiatric Association Publishing.

Borgatta, E., Boguslaw, R. & Haskell, M. (1976). On the work of Jacob L. Moreno. *Sociometry*, 38, 148–161.

Hare, A. & Hare, J. (1996). *J. L. Moreno*. London: Sage.

Jennings, H. H. (1943). *Leadership and isolation*. New York: Longman, Green and Co.

Lebovici, Serge. (1956). Psychoanalytical group psychotherapy. *Group Psychotherapy*, 9, 282–289.

Marineau, R. (1989). *Jacob Levy Moreno, 1889–1974*. New York: Routledge.

Moreno, J. D. (1989). Introduction. *Group Psychotherapy, Psychodrama & Group Psychotherapy*, 42, 3–12.

Moreno, J. L. (1920). *Das Testament des Vaters* [The words of the Father]. Berlin-Potsdam: Kiepenheuer Verlag.

Moreno, J. L. (1932). *In collaboration with E. S. Whitin Application of the group method to classification*. New York: National Committee on Prisons and Prison Labor.

Moreno, J. L. (1934). *Who shall survive? A new approach to the problems of human interrelations*. Washington, DC: Nervous and Mental Disease Publishing Company.

Moreno, J. L. (1947a). Open letter to group psychotherapists. *Sociatry*, 1, 16–30.

Moreno, J. L. (1947b). *The theater of spontaneity* (translated and revised from Das Stegreiftheater, 1923). Beacon, NY: Beacon House.

Moreno, J. L. (1953a). Preludes of the sociometric movement. In J. L. Moreno. *Who shall survive?* Beacon, NY: Beacon House. 13–108.

Moreno, J. L. (1953b). *Who shall survive?* Beacon, NY: Beacon House.

Moreno, J. L. (1955). The birth of a new era for sociometry. *Sociometry*, 18, 5–12.

Moreno, J. L. (1957). *The first book on group psychotherapy* (3rd Edition). Beacon, NY: Beacon House.

Moreno, J. L. (1989a). The autobiography of J. L. Moreno, M. D. (Abridged). *Group Psychotherapy, Psychodrama & Sociometry*, 42, 3–52.

Moreno, J. L. (1989b). The autobiography of J. L. Moreno, M. D. (Abridged) Part 2. *Group Psychotherapy, Psychodrama & Sociometry*, 42, 59–125.

Wampold, B. (2001). *The great psychotherapy debate*. Mahwah, NJ: Lawrence Erlbaum Associates.

INDEX